HEART
of the
JOURNEY

HEART
of the
JOURNEY

A Life of Adventure and Achievement,
With Three Days Mysteriously Lost to Time

JOHN BAKER

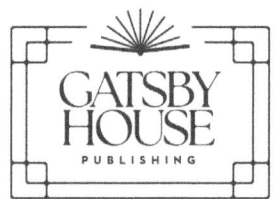

Copyright © 2025 by John Baker.

All rights reserved.

No part of this book may be reproduced in any form or by any electronic or mechanical means, including information storage and retrieval systems, without written permission from the author, except for the use of brief quotations in a book review.

This work is non-fiction and, as such, reflects the author's memory of his experiences. Many of the names and identifying characteristics of the individuals featured in this book have been changed to protect their privacy and certain individuals are composites. Dialogue and events have been recreated; in some cases, conversations have been edited to convey their substance rather than written exactly as they occurred.

ISBN: 979-8-9930129-3-3 (ebook)

ISBN: 979-8-9930129-2-6 (paperback)

ISBN: 979-8-9930129-4-0 (hardback)

Published in association with Gatsby House

www.gatsbyhousebooks.com

Dedication

To Margaret
aka Peggy

You have shown me the true essence of having a life partner.

Preface

Time is our most valuable asset and the only true nonrenewable resource. It continually moves forward. Once it's used, it's gone forever. I've been known to say, "This life isn't the dress rehearsal—it's the real thing." That feels truer now more than ever. It's a reminder that life is happening right now, and there's no second chance to live it. Every moment counts, urging us to live with intention and purpose. It's true what they say: *Time is precious.*

As you will see, I had three days tragically taken from me, and I was determined to reclaim them back . . . and then some. During my long recovery, I was granted a rare gift: the time to process, to be grateful, to write, and to live, but most of all to try to process how my near-death experience would change me. With that time, I was also able to fulfill a lifelong dream—to preserve the memories of my life I feared might one day fade.

This book is the result. It doesn't unfold in a straight line. Instead, my life-threatening incident weaves through the narrative, serving as the through line, with a series of flashbacks offering stories from childhood, milestones in adulthood, and everything in between. These stories are varied and, I believe, emotionally resonant. They reflect not just bold adventures, both in work and play, but a mindset—a zest for life, a willingness to face discomfort, and the drive to grow from it.

The following chapters are my story. Read it in one sitting or dip into it in pieces. If you decide not to read it at all, that's okay, too. At the very least, indulge me by reading Blair's foreword.

John Baker, 2025

Foreword

by Blair Baker

*A son is a son until he takes a wife,
but a daughter is a daughter all her life.*
—Irish proverb

Every phone call, before it's answered, has infinite possibilities. Like Schrödinger's cat, the phone call is everything and nothing until you press the phone to your ear. Of the calls we receive, very few are life-changing. On April 26, 2024, I received a call from my mom that did change my life: "Your dad's in the hospital. They don't know what's going on, but he is septic." Questions flashed through my mind: Septic? *What does that mean? How sick is he? Is my dad going to die?* Mortality is not a comfortable concept; it's filled with questions without answers that have plagued humans for generations. As a twenty-six-year-old with healthy parents, I'd only considered their deaths in infrequent nightmares, but in that moment, I was confronted with a most uncomfortable possibility: *Was I going to lose a parent?*

    Thankfully, as I'm sure you have surmised, because he is the author of this book, my dad lived. I didn't have to deal with the incredible sorrow of losing a parent, figuring out how to wade through day-to-day life with the indescribable grief of death. But what I was left with was emotional whiplash. When, several days later, it became clear my dad was going to survive, I was filled with joy, gratitude, and relief. An uncontrolled smile spread from the curves of my lips to my eyes.

Although I could let go of the imminent fear of my father's death, trauma doesn't just go away. It exists in me, even today, almost a year after that call from my mom. It exists each time I get a call from my parents, when my first thought is that something is wrong. It exists when I'm trying to fall asleep and the memories of his body in a hospital bed, on intensive life support, seep into my mind. It exists with each bug bite or tickle in my throat. Luckily, as these fears fade each day, I am left with another side effect: an appreciation for life and those I love, especially my dad.

My dad and I have always been close. While he worked growing up and my mom stayed at home to raise me and my brothers, my childhood memories with my dad are filled with vibrant child giggles and nights spent snuggling up to his chest for story time. His best stories weren't the ones he read from books, although we have a few family favorites. They were the stories he created himself, made up for me and my brothers. When I think about it, I can still feel the bright sun of an Idaho spring warming my face as we all scrambled onto the hammock, the breeze gently rocking us. As he started to speak, we were transported into another world. We followed *The Day in the Life of a Penny*, transported as it fell from the pocket of a busy businessman and landed heads-up, only to be picked up by a woman down on her luck. *The Flying Cow* took us across the country, showing us the vast array of landscapes the world has to offer, and *The Talking Dog* brought our childhood pets to life. His stories filled our imaginations, expanding the world of our small hometown into a much greater world, full of infinite universes for us to explore.

While many parents read to their kids, he created limitless adventures for us. Beyond the stories, he took the time to play with us. Nightly tickle fights ended with all of us in a heap of fitful giggles. A favorite tradition was building an elaborate fort made of cardboard boxes together called "Fort Maze." We would spend hours every night crafting second floors and slides out of what was in the local recycling bin, my dad using his architecture degree to turn a pile of cardboard into an elaborate fortress. He would squeeze his body into the smallest of child-size spaces, making a playground of our creation. His superpower—and for a kid, it was a literal superpower—was changing our reality to make it match our vibrant imaginations.

Heart of the Journey

As I've grown up and become an adult, our connection has remained close. Although I no longer need bedtime stories, ours is still a relationship of storytelling. We discuss politics, hobbies, friendships, the meanings of life, and the questions that fill our minds. It is no longer just him telling the stories; we share, weaving together our experiences, learning, and growing. While we may no longer build forts out of boxes, we still find ways to play and explore. We try new restaurants, travel around the world, and find the same joy we did when I was growing up. Beyond a parent, expert storyteller, and box-fort-maker, he became a friend.

Life is fragile. As you'll read in this book, innumerable factors led to his unlikely survival. The amazing hospital staff, the advancements of modern medicine, his already healthy body, and the support of loved ones led to the best gift I've ever received: his life. Although we were already close, this event strengthened the love we share. While we still chat about many of the same things, my dad's incident took our relationship to another level with a desire to engage more deeply in each other's lives. I choose to go home on my vacation days and spend afternoons together on the golf course because those are the moments I almost lost. And it's those moments that I cherish the most.

Through it all, I have become more loving and appreciative not just of my dad but everyone in my life and so has he. He is still the same person at his core—even in the hospital, he was checking stock prices and asking about the news—but I have seen his heart soften. His love for those around him has expanded. It's not just something I've experienced through more frequent calls and tighter hugs. More than anything, I felt it: His energy has shifted. You can see in his eyes the genuine warmth and appreciation for those that he loves. His story could easily fill your mind with fear of the unpredictable, but I hope you take away the same conclusion that he has of loving deeper, loving more, and loving louder. You never know what curveballs life is going to throw your way, but hopefully, no matter what happens, you have a supportive community of family and friends to walk the journey with you. After all, it's the people around you who make life worth living.

Table of Contents

Introduction: Three Lost Days 1

1. The ER 4
2. Overcoming Fears 10
3. Tuesday Morning Swim 18
4. Signs of Trouble 21
5. An Uncomfortable Flight 25

6. Roots in San Francisco 32
7. Golden Days 41
8. Learning My Own Way 45
9. An Italian Adventure 52
10. New Zealand Awaits 63
11. Early Years as a GC 68

12. Code Blue 75
13. The Battle Begins 78
14. In the Deep 84
15. Seven Missed Calls 88

16. Building More Than Dreams 93
17. Tin Cup (The Town, Not the Movie) 100

Photos I..108

18. Avalanche...125

19. Crossroads..129
20. A Curious Case 134

21. Vail Beginnings 137
22. Putting Down Roots 143
23. Lessons in Life Balance.....................................148
24. Terry 153

25. The Waiting Game 157

26. Our Early Sun Valley Years...............................166
27. Family Fun and Fort Maze 178

Photos II 187

28. Career Opportunities 202
29. Deals and Diversification..................................211
30. Quiet Chaos...217

31. Saint Sophia 223
32. Long Road Back 229
33. Life Saga...241

Acknowledgments..252
About the Authors...255

Introduction

Three Lost Days

I am here because you were there.

—Dara Torres

Memories are tricky. Unless you're that rare person who has a photographic memory, your mind can't hold everything that's ever happened to you. Details slip away like losing your cell phone in the bed linens: you put your phone down for just a moment, and the next thing you know, you're patting around the sheets, trying to locate what should be an easy-to-find object. And if you're lucky, someone will be beside you, prodding at the sheets, too.

Often, all it takes to bring a memory to the forefront is a word or phrase that sparks the recollection, just like pulling back the right part of the sheets to reveal where your phone was all along.

Then there are times when memories cease to exist. You frantically run through the library of your thoughts, but the metaphorical book you're looking for isn't on any of the shelves. No matter how many times someone jogs your memory, there's nothing but a dark, empty well where remembrance should be. That's one of the most helpless feelings a person can have. Your mind has betrayed you or is hiding the events you so desperately want to remember.

I know a little something about feeling powerless while trying to recall something. There are three days in April 2024 that I cannot remember.

John Baker

From April 26 to 29, I couldn't, and still can't, recall what happened to me—not if my life depended on it, which is unfortunate, because my life had truly hung in the balance on those days. This gap in my memory is a by-product of an experience that left a deep imprint on my life. Even the couple of days on either side of that mental black hole are like looking at an old, half-developed, and full-on faded Polaroid. I can make out the shape and outline of those events, but I cannot always drill down to exact details.

To piece together the end of a picture-perfect Hawaiian getaway that ended with being checked into an ER in San Francisco, I have relied heavily on the people who saved my life. The primary eyewitnesses I've leaned on are my wife Peggy, my children, and several medical professionals, including my cardiologist Dr. David Daniels and lifelong friend Dr. Peter Callander. If it were not for them, I wouldn't be here to tell my story. I'm eternally grateful to them and to everyone else who contributed to my care, and you'll see in the following pages how they impacted my life.

Of course, writing a memoir when you can't remember three important days of your life presents a challenge, but I do not doubt that the reports I've received from my friends and family are 100 percent accurate. According to them, the solution was to write this book in a first-person perspective for a cohesive read, braiding timelines between the ER and my early days, and adding details as they were told to me to fill in the blanks.

Those three lost days changed many things. They reframed the way I see the world, my family, and myself. Yet even in the fog of what I can't recall, the lessons I learned from that period are crystal clear. This book is not just about those lost days or even the events surrounding them. It's about the bigger picture—about resilience, the human capacity for adaptation, and the raw determination it takes to turn disaster into triumph. It's a book about an individual who had unknowingly been preparing his whole life to overcome just such a tragedy, and a story of how the spirit can keep going even when the mind and body try to shut down. Could such an ordeal leave one's perspective on life untouched? Not a chance.

It's also a lesson for those who feel helpless in the hands of a medical system that is sometimes seemingly rigid. For those who have attended medical school, there's a saying that most likely comes up here: "When you hear hoofbeats, think horses, not zebras." It's a medical adage used to rein in physicians' diagnoses. It means: When diagnosing, doctors should first consider the most probable common explanations of a patient's symptoms (hoofbeats = horses) before jumping to rare or exotic conditions (the so-called "zebras"). In other words, the most straightforward explanation is usually correct. That works wonderfully if you're about to be trampled by a herd of horses, but I had been faced with a zebra. Telling a doctor with gobs of training and expertise that what they're doing just isn't working for you takes courage. It takes discussing your symptoms openly, even when they don't fit the textbook description or seem relevant. Sometimes, you or your loved ones must insist on more tests, second opinions, and alternative treatments.

The final takeaway from my story is that a fear of what could happen is no reason not to seek adventure. Dozens of people who have heard my story have asked if I regretted swimming in wide-open waters or wished that I had ditched my regular Hawaiian morning ocean swim for a much safer dip in the neighboring lap pool. But there's not a single thing I'd change, including the event that changed my life forever.

Missing out on life because "something bad might happen" is a boring way to live. Life equates to risk. You cannot leave your house without the chance of something bad happening; you could also be sitting on your sofa and a meteor could come crashing through your ceiling. (That actually happened to an Alabama woman in 1954.) Life is meant to be experienced. And on the other side of a second chance at life, I fully intend to experience everything I can.

With all that in mind, I invite you to walk with me through this story not as a passive observer but as a fellow traveler. There's value in the journey, even if your grand adventures have more than their share of misfortunes. It's in the highs and lows that we learn how to deal with life's successes and failures. You need the lows to appreciate the views from the top. By the end, I hope you'll see a path forward for the obstacles in life as I have in mine. Even when the risks are unclear or forgotten or the outcome is wildly unexpected, taking the road less traveled is always worth the journey.

1

The ER

The trouble with trouble is it starts out as fun.
—Mark Twain

April 26, 2024, Friday

2:00 a.m. on a Friday morning is not a great time to be admitted to a San Francisco emergency room. Thursday nights are party nights for many college kids, and alcohol-induced injuries abound. San Francisco's unhoused population is at crisis levels, and those folks, like the man humming "Hotel California" while clutching his ripped-up shirt, have no other place to go for medical or mental health care.

Then there's the staff. Every doctor and nurse in the place looks as fresh-faced as Doogie Howser. If there's a seasoned doctor to be found in the halls, they're only there because they drew the short straw for the overnight shift. No one wants to be there, my wife Peggy and me included.

A few minutes earlier, we'd been picked up by an Uber at our hotel and deposited unceremoniously at the ER entrance of California Pacific Medical Center (CPMC) Van Ness Campus. I wouldn't have called for a ride under normal circumstances. I would have preferred walking straight up Geary Street to Van Ness Avenue, passing Union Square. The once-vibrant public plaza was one of San Francisco's cultural hubs known for high-end retail stores, art galleries, and theaters. I doubted the dress code for any of those places included the slippers I was wearing—even if they did sport the Four Seasons logo. I'd been able to get myself dressed, my shirt tucked in with a belt, but I'd forgotten to put on my shoes when we left our room. To be fair, I was already in the early stages of multiorgan system failure, but no one knew that yet.

There were signs, however. Just thirty minutes earlier, I'd used our bathroom at the hotel and, looking in the bowl afterward, wondered why my urine was brown. That couldn't be good.

When the Uber arrived at the ER entrance, I was able to get out of the vehicle on my own, although cautiously and slowly. While I was technically awake and ambulatory, I was mentally checked out. I wasn't even coherent enough to have an adequate amount of fear or concern over my situation. I barely remember shuffling past the smokers, the ones who can be found standing outside the entrance of any ER, hoping the nicotine will soothe their nerves.

As I followed Peggy inside, I was directed to sit in a chair with an ottoman in the waiting room while she went into action, checking me in and filling out the necessary forms. My wife explained to the medical staff what was going on but not what had happened. That's because neither she nor I knew exactly what had happened. Regardless, the hospital admissions person was less interested in what was going on than in verifying that I had decent insurance.

While Peggy was able to communicate with the staff at the front desk, the ones wearing face masks presented a problem. Most people are unaware of my wife's hearing impairment, a condition she's managed since birth—only the most observant might catch the subtle signs of a slight speech impediment or what some interpret as an "accent." She's an exceptional lip reader, but face masks render that gift useless. In moments like that, Peggy will normally glance at me, and I'm always nearby, ready to translate without her needing to ask. But this time, I wasn't there to help.

I've never seen her hearing impairment as a limitation. To me, it's something distinctive, almost like a superpower—granting her heightened perception and extraordinary organizational skills. She was calling on both of those powers in that moment, as she stepped forward to advocate for my care.

The waiting room was modern and presentable, since the hospital was only four years old. But a hospital next to the Tenderloin, notoriously the roughest neighborhood in San Francisco, can only be so clean. As my wife filled out paperwork, I made myself at home and propped my feet up on the ottoman. By now, my right ankle was swollen, sore, and blistered. Blood was visibly collecting under the tissue.

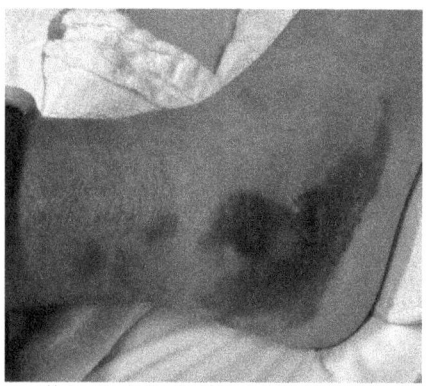

Swelling and signs of trouble on the plane

The admissions person looked past Peggy and yelled to me, "Baby, that's contaminated with germs—don't touch that thing." I did as I was told. Given what was happening with my foot, more germs were the last thing I needed.

As soon as Peggy finished filling out the paperwork, we were told a triage nurse would come get me in a few minutes. Time was an abstraction to me. We could have been sitting in that microcosm of humanity for five minutes or five years. The people around me led diverse lives that intersected at the crisis points of vulnerability and urgency. From someone who had just come from the Four Seasons to the unhoused person sitting in the corner, we were all bound together by the shared need for care.

Right after I was checked in, a mother brought in a little girl, a toddler. There wasn't anything visibly wrong with her, but for someone so young to be in an ER at zero dark thirty, it couldn't have been good. The girl and her mom went through the same rigamarole we did, but the little girl was taken to triage first. "We'll get to you in just a minute," the triage nurse said to Peggy and me.

We sat and were patient, because that's what you do. While the ER provides the actual treatment, staffed by qualified medical professionals with specialized training and equipment, the triage team quickly assesses and determines the urgency and order of care. Sure enough, it was only a few more long minutes until a male triage nurse came back for me. I was then run through the usual battery of diagnostics—my pulse, blood pressure, temperature, and pupil dilation all got checked, and he also took a blood sample. He said little, seeming to be running on autopilot. It would have been nice if he had shared with Peggy that my temperature was elevated, and my blood pressure was on the low end of acceptable, but we wouldn't be given any more feedback or test results for another hour.

We left the triage room after twenty minutes and were sent back out to the waiting area for another twenty until a nurse arrived. She told us we would be moving to a pediatric waiting room, because two cardiac patients had just been brought into the adult side and they wanted to give us a quieter space. As we were being led down a hallway away from urgent care, I felt vaguely insignificant. The drab colors of the adult ER had been transformed into festive, kid-friendly décor, but the perceived demotion in care status didn't do our hearts any good. We just wanted to know what was wrong with me, and no one besides us seemed to be interested in finding out.

I ended up in a room right next door to the toddler who'd arrived after us. Had I been more with it, I would have thought about our children. If you're a parent, you can't help but take on a little of the pain for a sick child. Peggy would have been more empathetic about everyone else in the hospital had we been visiting a sick friend. As it was, she was exhausted. She'd been dealing with me all day, on top of traveling from Hawaii and researching Bay Area ERs for the entire flight.

After a while, I felt the urge to use the restroom again. A nurse gave me a cup to urinate in before she disappeared. This time around, the liquid was an even deeper shade of orange-brown, a color that was nowhere near normal. *How is it even darker than before?* I wondered.

At that, Peggy walked into the hall to find help. "The doctor is in the next room and will visit your room next," a nurse explained.

That's when my frustrated wife bent her ear. "His urine is brown. Aren't you going to give him an IV or something? He needs fluids, doesn't he?" She was told a doctor would have to order an IV. The nurse at least agreed to grab a warming blanket for me.

Meanwhile, my foot was still a dark purple hue and had continued to blister even more than before. There was no doubt now that my swollen ankle was the color of royalty.

We sat there for another half an hour before a measured voice came over the intercom, relaying information in the esoteric codes and phrases of hospital-speak. Between that and the cross-chatter we were picking up from the ER staff running through the halls, Peggy figured out that one of the cardiac patients had coded. Keep in mind that there are at least three other medical emergency facilities within a five-mile radius of where we were; to bring two heart attacks to an ER that looked like it was already at capacity must have meant the City by the Bay had a lot of sick people that night.

From time to time, Peggy would rest her head on my hospital bed and close her eyes only to be startled awake by the slightest movement. Had I been in my right mind, I would have urged her to go find a quieter place to rest; there was nothing to do until a doctor saw me. But I'm glad she stayed by my side.

Amid all the chaos in the hallways, I experienced a moment of alertness and told her I was in pain. She again flagged down a nurse who passed by the room, telling her the same thing she'd said to the previous nurse: "He needs fluids." This time, the result was more favorable.

A few minutes later, the nurse returned with an IV bag along with some antibiotics to administer through it. With a little boost of saline in my system, I'd surely be on the mend. Maybe I'd perk up enough so that Peggy could get some sleep. Maybe I could relax enough to get some sleep, too. With the IV in place, my eyes soon felt heavy, and then I was out.

Except I didn't take a light nap. I had full-blown passed out.

Thankfully, the nurse was right there in the room, covering me with warm blankets when I went pale and my eyes rolled back.

"Honey. Honey. Honey!" Peggy shouted while shaking me. The nurse shook me, too, searching for a pulse. Not finding one and with no response, the nurse hit the code button and started chest compressions. Peggy ran toward the nurses' station, shouting, "Help, help! He's passed out! He's coding! We need help!"

At least ten medical staff rushed in from all directions, one of them instinctively grabbing a crash cart along the way. Peggy stood in the hall terrified, watching it all unfold, listening to the beeps and whirs of the life-giving machines. More medical staff checked my pulse in a few different places, but they still couldn't find one. The conversation and actions among the medical team grew more urgent. Peggy could do nothing but watch.

I can't imagine what I would have felt if the script had been flipped, and I'd had to watch my helpless, lifeless wife in a hospital bed as a nurse called over the intercom: "*Code blue, code blue in Pediatrics, code blue.*"

I can't imagine, but Peggy can.

2

Overcoming Fears

The only thing we have to fear is fear itself.
—FDR

There is no place on the planet like Hawaii. Emerald, mist-wrapped mountains rise from the ocean's depths and are platforms for cascading waterfalls that carve verdant valleys. It's as if nature herself had been painting a masterpiece to appeal to all the human senses. The air is sweet with the scent of plumeria—the flowers used to make leis. Almost everywhere you go, the rhythmic hum of the waves creates a symphony that soothes the soul. Time slows, and your worries seem to dissolve.

With every sunrise or sunset, the sky blazes in hues of orange, pink, and violet that warm the skin and heal the heart. Out of the rich volcanic soil grow sugar, pineapple, coffee, and macadamia nuts, Hawaiian staples that offer the world a taste of the islands' bounty and provide an ideal landscape for bees to pollinate and gather nectar. In Hawaii, paradise isn't just a word; it's a lifestyle, a feeling that stays with you every day you're there. It's why Peggy and I started spending more time on Hawaii's Kohala Coast years ago.

Our three children were still young, and we wanted a new location for family activity and adventure while being able to slow down at the same time. That sounds oxymoronic unless you've lived in Hawaii a while. You can't go through a single day on the islands without being presented with a healthy opportunity to swim in the ocean, outrigger canoe, prone board, stand-up paddle, or play tennis or golf. The islands cater to those who seek out physical activity in paradise.

Our beautiful Hawaiian home provided the balance we had been searching for throughout our entire married lives. I'd worked hard for decades building a successful commercial real estate business, and together, we had been managing various public and private investments. Now, we were at an age and of a mindset that we still wanted to work hard, but we wanted to play hard as well. Still, splitting our time between Hawaii and the mainland fulfilled all those needs.

The "work hard" part of that equation wasn't difficult to pull off—we'd filled our lives with work and family. It was the "play hard" aspect that had to be planned for. It was easy to get sucked into this deal or that conference call, or into board positions that required us to be available in different time zones. I had to remind myself that adventure and travel were at the core of who I am and who I always had been. That sense of adventure had been passed down to me by my parents, who valued nature and an active lifestyle. It's a gift that continues to shape my life—especially in my marriage, where Peggy and I share those values.

I've been active my entire life in one form or another, whether as an avid climber, a marathon runner, a mountain biker, or a swimmer. I recall a friend patting me on the back once to congratulate me on the discipline it took to keep fit enough to do all those activities. I graciously accepted the compliment and thought about what they didn't know: Two of my sporting pursuits, rock climbing and swimming, were chosen specifically to confront my fears of heights and water.

In the summer of 2013, I was introduced to rock climbing by my friend Thomas Laffont. He had recently spent time scaling some of the nearby rock faces in the Jackson Hole area and had shared some pictures of the highlights with me. In one of the images, he was propped up high on a knoll with the sun in his face, the Tetons sloping away behind him like something out of a movie. I could tell his smile was authentic—it showed a true sense of accomplishment, and my interest was piqued as I took it all in. There was added comfort in knowing that he had hired an experienced guide. Soon after, we started planning for our own multiday climb in the Tetons' backcountry, preparing to scale Mount Moran's granite face outside Jackson, Wyoming.

Thomas rattled off gear lists and logistics while I scribbled notes, my pulse quickening with every detail. Then, he paused and said, almost offhandedly, "There will be times during the climb when things get a bit airy." He let the words hang there, like he was testing whether I truly understood.

"Airy," I repeated, not sure whether I should laugh or worry.

He nodded. "It means you're high up, maybe exposed, nothing but space on one side. And there's this one spot," he added, lowering his voice a little, "where we actually have to rappel down—*midway* through the climb. And in the dark, before the sun even rises."

I swallowed hard, picturing myself dangling in blackness, the beam of my headlamp bouncing off sheer rock with only a rope and my trust in Thomas keeping me from the void. But I had learned early on in climbing that there were times when the option of turning back was simply no longer an option—it was how you got over your fear of heights, I guess.

***

Water remains one of my most enduring fears, one that still haunts me to this day. That particular phobia came into my life twofold. The first part came about while playing around with friends in my grandparents' swimming pool in Marin County as a kid. There was a friend of mine—who I'm sure I'd been pestering to within an inch of his sanity, though I can't quite remember the circumstances that led up to him dunking my head underwater. As his hand pushed down on the back of my head, plunging me under the cold water, my lungs felt like they were going to burst as I struggled to break free. The whole thing might have lasted five seconds, but it felt like eternity. I was convinced I was going to die right there—and the fear of drowning followed me around in all the years that followed. That fear didn't keep me out of the water completely, but I've noticed myself being more cautious when diving into the deep end of a pool, or when swimming in the ocean, later in life.

The second part, which certainly didn't help my fear of water, was watching the iconic movie *Jaws* when it debuted in June 1975. Like most twelve-year-olds, I was heavily impressionable, and those scenes of bloody massacres created a lingering sense of unease in me (and most beachgoers, at the time). That mechanical shark, the first of its kind, became a symbol of fear itself. It represented the dark and mysterious forces that could disrupt our lives when we least expected it. At such a young age, I associated any body of water—ocean and pool alike—with fear.

Thankfully, there were some positive influences in my late teens when it came to the water. I recall observing my grandmother Virginia Baker swimming in the fifteen-meter pool at the Royal Towers apartments in San Francisco. Visible through the fog, her swimming appeared to be almost effortless, her rhythmic breaststroke creating a peaceful tempo as she glided through the water. It felt somewhat surreal: She was swimming alone in the cool, brisk air, simply enjoying the peaceful exercise. I admired how natural and at ease she looked in the water.

Still, my fear of drowning has been one of the paradoxical attractions to spending extended periods of time on an island surrounded by water. Similar to my initial fear of rock climbing, I knew that the only way through that fear was to confront it head-on. So, I chose to make swimming an intentional and consistent part of my weekly routine.

It certainly helps that our community in Hawaii has beachfront access and encourages friendly participation in all sports that might get your hair wet. The emphasis on water sports means that pretty much any time I want to swim in the ocean or do any other aquatic activity, I'm not alone. I am always under the watchful eye of a waterman.

A waterman is someone highly skilled and comfortable in the water. They often excel in a variety of ocean-related activities and embody a lifestyle that revolves around the water. To Hawaiians, being a waterman is more than just being good at water sports—it's about having a deep respect and connection to the ocean, to nature, and to both of their rhythms. Watermen can educate and offer comfort to anyone new to ocean sports.

They are often seen not just as protectors of those who participate in aquatic activities but as spiritual guardians of the sea itself. To always have a practiced waterman watching my back while I was in the ocean has been a game changer for me. They have been a safety net that has helped me address my fears on my own terms.

When I first started ocean swimming, I had to use fins to keep up with the other swimmers in the group and to provide my own method of risk management. In open water, the swells can batter you from every angle—micro tides swirl for no discernable reason and throw off your stroke. But if disaster struck, I figured the fins would offer some sense of security. No one teased or belittled me for using them. Everyone accepted that no matter the water sport, we all started at different levels; what counted was trying your best and finishing with a smile. The positive peer pressure of a group was what I needed to push me over the top.

To this day, the fellow swimmers in my group are encouraging and always genuinely glad to see me down at the beach, ready to swim. After we catch up for a few minutes, we hit the water in the large bay bordering our community's beachfront, where there is a buoy about a half mile out. The bay is perfect for any number of water sports. Whether fishing or paddle boarding, there is always someone out there, enjoying the ocean. It was as safe as anywhere in the ocean could be—until the day it wasn't.

In the spring of 2018, a father and son were stand-up paddleboarding in the bay. They were no more than 150 yards offshore, in water twenty-five feet deep—that's kiddie pool depth, for the ocean. The pair were minding their own business when a twelve-foot tiger shark decided the son's paddleboard was a big fish. The shark knocked the young man off his board and attacked, lacerating his right forearm and hand and, worst of all, taking his right leg off below the knee. After attacking the son, the tiger shark turned toward Dad before it eventually swam off.

All the work I'd done to overcome my fear of water evaporated once I heard that news. A number of folks in the swimming group rightfully said, "Hey, that's too risky. I respect the ocean, but I'm not going out into open waters anymore."

Heart of the Journey

I was one of those people. I stayed away from the ocean for several years. I'd do laps in the pool, but it was nothing like the earlier commitment I'd made to swimming in the ocean a few times a week. I wasn't yet ready to confront my fear head-on once more. I wasn't sure I'd ever feel up to ocean swimming again.

What my fellow watermen in Hawaii didn't know was that I'd had a shark encounter of my own, many years before—in 2004, while scuba diving with Peggy's father and a few other friends. Our group had been spearfishing off the coast of St. Martin, and we'd just speared a large grouper when an aggressive shark came by to see what all the commotion was about. I watched as the shark swam behind my scuba partner and nudged her hard in the back. As the shark turned toward me, I started swimming backward and screamed "F—k," losing the regulator from my mouth. Then, I had to make a quick decision: shoot my spear gun at the oncoming Jaws-lookalike or pay the possible consequences.

My arrow narrowly missed the creature's nose, grazing the side of its right dorsal fin. It bolted over to the other swimmers, who had seen what was going on and were gathered on a rock outcropping on the ocean floor next to the divemaster. The divemaster wisely tossed our bag of smaller fish in front of the circling shark, distracting it from the scuba group. My last clear visual of the shark was seeing it grab the sack of bloody fish and swim off into the murky water, never to be seen again. As it disappeared, it shook its head—maybe to get a better grip or out of irritation, like it hadn't gotten exactly what it wanted.

It had taken me over a decade to overcome that incident and to feel comfortable enough to swim in Hawaii's waters. Then, with the awful attack on the boy, my fears had returned in full force.

***

At sixty, swimming means more to me now than it ever has. I'd always carried the idea that I should learn to swim—maybe to finally move past my childhood fear of water, or maybe because I sensed it could be a sport that would keep me fit well into my later years.

John Baker

Back in 2009, at age forty-five, I would watch the lap swimmers at Zenergy, Sun Valley's health and swim club, with a mix of admiration and envy. That's where I decided to make a change—a small decision that became a turning point in my athletic life. I decided to start swimming laps in the indoor pool, avoiding the six-lane outdoor lap pool where the masters swim class trained.

From my side of the glass, I'd watch them and wonder: *How do they stay on the surface so effortlessly? How can they swim for so long? And those flip turns, they look so pro—how do you even learn that?* Wearing my board shorts, no swim cap, and awkward, oversized goggles, I'd study their smooth strokes and speed, marveling at the flow that made them look like Olympians. In fact, one of them was—Dara Torres, a twelve-time Olympic medalist and local hero. At forty-one, she became the oldest person to earn a spot on the 2008 U.S. Olympic Swim Team, and she'd occasionally drop in for a swim, making the whole scene even more inspiring.

I was captivated by their elegant form and the precision of each stroke. I knew that if I committed myself, I could overcome my fear of water, learn to float effortlessly, and maybe even master a flip turn. In 2010, my friend and disciplined swimming pal, Katherine McGowan, took the time to teach me the basics, while Maria Beattie—patient, encouraging, and with the swim talent to back it up—coached from the deck.

As I neared the wall, I'd keep my hands at my sides and tuck my chin into my chest. Then came the bend of my knees, the roll underwater, and planting my feet flat against the wall. After a strong push-off and an underwater breaststroke, my head would break the surface for a breath. It sounds seamless now, but in the beginning, it was anything but—instead, it was hundreds of failed attempts, with water shooting up my nose and more than a few kick-offs that had me surfacing in the wrong lane entirely.

But persistence paid off. After a month of practice, I nailed the turn and began to feel like a "real swimmer." From there, I worked steadily on my strokes, breathing, and endurance. Over the next decade, those efforts carried me into the outdoor masters' pool, where I swam alongside the people I had once only watched from a distance. With Maria's gentle persistence, I eventually traded my board shorts for streamlined jammers, added a swim cap, and wore proper goggles that stayed put during that now-fluid underwater turn.

***

The hardcore members of my Hawaii swim group respectfully worked on me for several years after the 2018 Hawaii shark incident, trying to get me back into the water—but just because one of my core tenets is facing my fears through action, that doesn't mean I climbed the mountain in one step.

Fortunately, personal challenges and positive peer pressure have always been a whirlwind of motivation for me. I did eventually get back in the ocean, little by little. I'd swim out to a point where my paranoia would get the best of me, and I'd "*Nope*" my way back to shore. It was embarrassing that when a piece of seaweed or another swimmer brushed against my leg, I'd flinch; if I felt anything more than the water on my skin, I'd become convinced I was Jaws' next meal and panic-paddle back to shore, eventually laughing about it once I'd regulated my breathing and heart rate.

We emphasize what's crucial in our lives. For me, I knew that meant eventually setting the fear aside and getting back to where I was before the shark attack. This took time, intention, and positive self-talk. But, little by little, I made progress until I was fully back to my deep-water ways.

3

Tuesday Morning Swim

Calm rarely sends a warning before the storm.
—ChatGPT

April 23, 2024, Tuesday (three days earlier)

On workout mornings in Hawaii, my alarm typically went off by 6:00 a.m.—usually before Peggy stirred. I'd shuffle into the kitchen and start the coffee or tea, whichever called to me first. With a glass of electrolyte-infused water in my other hand, I sank into my favorite chair, the remote already waiting. Since Hawaii is three hours behind our hometown in Idaho, getting up that early gave me a chance to catch up on any significant work updates from the mainland. My reasonably peaceful morning routine allowed me to respond to a dozen emails and texts within fifteen to twenty minutes while enjoying my beverages.

Two or three times a week, by ten minutes to seven, I'd cruise down to the beach in a golf cart, waving to neighbors out walking dogs or just enjoying their coffee. "Water looks good today," someone would call out. After checking the swell and tossing out a few light jokes about murky water, we'd slip on our goggles and head for the morning mile.

We'd finish the swim around ten minutes to eight. I'd trade a few parting words with the crew and then head to the beach bar, sand still on my ankles. Then, I might have another coffee or just some berries and yogurt—that was a ritual all its own. By the time I returned, Peggy would be in her element, checking emails, trading stock options, or chatting with our kids on the phone (and often all at once): "No, Wilson, I'm telling you—celery juice is the secret . . ."

For Peggy, morning consumption routines are a combination of whatever the top health experts are saying on how you should start the day. This includes drinking hot water with lemon juice, followed by celery juice, green tea, and a cappuccino with 2% milk—plus using a neti pot, if she's experiencing any allergies. We're all creatures of habit, to some extent; however, I love moderation, mixing things up, and knowing when to keep my mouth shut. When I got back from my swim, we'd catch up and talk about what we had planned for later that day. By nine, both of us were primed and ready to roll for the rest of the day.

That was our morning life in Hawaii—calm, predictable, and full of small pleasures—until Tuesday, April 23, 2024. My day started off like a fine Swiss timepiece. I was in the water on time and was a little more than halfway to the buoy by 7:15 a.m. Midstroke, I could see the swimmers on my right. I was trying to sense where the others were to keep a comfortable distance and avoid bumping into them.

I swam on until I felt it—an electric current passing through my lower body. I knew immediately I'd been stung. If you swim in the ocean long enough, you're going to get stung by a jellyfish, but the smart course of action in the open water is *not* to panic. Instead, you quickly assess the situation, then keep going until you get to safety.

The jellyfish stings I'd experienced in the past felt like getting zapped by a bee—painful, but nothing I couldn't handle. It shocks you, and you get immediate redness, swelling, and a raised welt at the site of the jab, but then it's gone in a day or two. But that wasn't how this particular situation unfolded.

In the water, I paused for a moment to self-assess, floating and treading water as I tried to make sense of what had happened. I didn't feel any residual pain, so I figured I was fine. It wasn't a shark nibble, after all.

The only thing that concerned me at all was the difference between this sting and the jellyfish stings I'd had before. With past stings, the pain could be pinpointed to the exact site, but this one felt like multiple barbs had pierced my skin at once. It was more electric jolt than surface pain. It was . . . curious. But with everyone else already on their way to the buoy, I knew I had to stay the course to avoid falling too far behind. I kicked into high gear and swam to the buoy, where we paused to regroup before continuing back to shore.

One of the guys with us that day was waterman Thibert (endearingly pronounced T-Bear). He's the quintessential Polynesian waterman, embracing Hawaiian life. In his late forties, this fellow is bronze and built. If ever there was an archetype of a waterman, he was it—he exudes an infectious calm. I always knew that if I were in trouble out there, T-Bear would be the guy to pull me out of the water—just like he and his team had during that shark attack several years earlier.

T-Bear is a "Don't worry about sharks unless you see a fin" kind of guy. I considered my sting a non-issue, so I chose not to share it with the group. That's how I treated it when I got back to shore as well. I didn't even bother mentioning it to Peggy when we linked back up after my swim, because in my mind, the sting, although different, was nothing more than a minor annoyance that sometimes occurs while enjoying time in the ocean, a footnote to a relatively routine day in paradise.

4

Signs of Trouble

Risks must be taken because the greatest hazard in life is to risk nothing.
—William Arthur Ward

April 24, 2024, Wednesday

We rarely get sick in Hawaii. I don't know what it is, but the environment doesn't lend itself to illness. I know that's as scientific sounding as a fortune cookie, but there's just something about the climate, clean air, healthy food, and laid-back lifestyle that seem to keep people feeling healthier. So, when I woke up Wednesday morning with a slight fever, I thought it was odd.

I tested positive for COVID-19 once in August 2023. Other than that, I can't remember the last time I was ill since the kids were still at home. I love my kids, but when they were younger, they were like little Petri dishes, passing around every cold or flu from their classmates as if it were a class project. To combat this, I became a firm believer that staying positive, active, and continuing with my usual routine would shake off any minor bugs with minimal symptoms in no time.

At 70°F with a slight ocean breeze, Wednesday had all the makings of a perfect day. I hadn't planned on an ocean swim, so I scheduled a pool session with a few buddies instead. Peggy was playing pickleball at 10:00 a.m., and I told her I'd catch up with her afterward. Aside from a low-grade fever and the dull headache that had lingered since the night before, the morning unfolded more or less as usual. It felt like many mornings before it—routine, familiar. Looking back, there were no clear warning signs, just a quiet sense that the day wasn't quite what it seemed.

After finishing my swim, I headed to the courts where Peggy and her friends were pickleballing. I sensed from her that it was a friendly game, but winning is always a matter of pride. The sun was on my face as I watched, hearing the *dink* of the ball and the laughter from the court. Then, a switch flipped inside me as those sounds faded from my mind. It was like I'd been teleported to the Arctic Circle. I don't think I had any visible shakes, but the waves of cold that were swirling through my body told a different story. I used to believe that being chilled to the bone was just some random expression people parroted when they were excessively cold. But at that moment, there were frozen fingers inside me, intent on touching every single bone in my body. The longer I stood watching Peggy play, the colder I got.

Peggy had improved so much that her matches were fun to observe, and usually, I would get comfortable and watch the competition unfold. Instead, I caught her attention between shots to say, "I'm heading back to the house."

"Why?" Peggy asked, confused.

"I'm not feeling well," I said flatly.

When Peggy arrived home shortly after I did, she went into mom mode, bringing me a rarely used thermometer. A moment later, there was a beep. My temperature was 100.7°F. *That's odd*, I thought. *How could I be sick?*

We were scheduled to fly out the following afternoon to San Francisco, where we'd spend the night in the city before we continued to Mexico on Friday morning. Peggy looked at the thermometer and then at me before she said, "You get some rest—here's some Advil."

I knew she was right. Something was off, and I knew I should listen to my body, so I canceled my plans for that day—which was odd for me. On the rare occasion that I feel off, I might take a quick nap or rest a bit before throwing in the towel on an entire day. Instead, I flushed the rest of my schedule with a few texts:

I'm sorry, I can't see you this afternoon. Maybe next time I'm in town.

A beer at the beach bar is out for tonight. Can't be helped. I'm so sorry.

I had just over a day left in Hawaii, and I wanted to squeeze every last drop out of the time I had left. Time with friends is irreplaceable, and I was still hoping to end the trip on a high note, but I could already tell I wasn't going to get all my boxes checked.

As I headed to the bedroom to lie down, I had an epiphany. At a dinner event on Monday night, I'd run into a guy who frequently participated in our morning swims. He was about my age and always gave me a run for my money in the water. He'd been coughing that night like he had a cold. *That must be it*, I thought. *I picked up a virus from him*. With that, I proudly told my wife that I'd Sherlock Holmesed my malady.

Peggy is the quintessential problem solver in the family, so for a moment, she became a human computer, merging facts and probabilities. She concluded that it couldn't possibly have come from my friend Monday night and pronounced, "It's something else."

Eh, what does she know? I thought. I just needed a little rest.

I followed the advice of another friend, Satoshi Nakajima, who adheres to a strict protocol of taking a nap while mummifying yourself in blankets when sick. The theory is that you'll sweat out the fever, and you'll be good in no time.

At noon, I came to, my phone blowing up with text messages:

Where are you?

What's going on?

Are you okay?

What the hell was going on? Through a slight mental fog, I remembered that my regular Wednesday golf game had been scheduled for high noon, but in the flurry of canceling plans, I'd forgotten to let the guys know my status. I was rarely late, so my buddies were rightly worried about me. I felt horrible that I'd let the guys down. After all, it was supposed to be the final round I had scheduled on the trip.

When I told Peggy I'd missed the golf game, she urged me to rest a bit longer. Lying in bed, I turned toward the windows and took in the view—lush tropical foliage, the shimmer of the ocean, and neighboring volcanoes rising in the distance. From the bedroom, you can hear the distant sound of waves crashing against the shore and feel the gentle breeze rustling through the palm trees. The sounds pulled me back under, and I drifted off again.

A few hours later, I woke up on my own, thankful that my phone wasn't blowing up with texts about other plans I'd forgotten to cancel. But when I went to the bathroom, I noticed my urine was uncharacteristically yellow. Once again, I consulted Peggy, the Problem Solver.

"You're likely dehydrated," she said. "Why don't you drink more water?"

I couldn't argue with the logic—chugging water often helped. With a fever, it made sense that I might need extra fluids, so I gulped down as much as I could. Unfortunately, hydration, I would later find out, was not the key to feeling any better.

I slugged around the house for the next few hours, finally deciding I'd like to try a quick bite at the beach bar with Peggy for dinner. It took all my strength to get there, and I realized I hadn't eaten much that day as Peggy had been administering me Advil and Tylenol.

At dinner, I kept my distance, trying not to expose anyone to whatever I had picked up. Afterward, we took the cart back to the house, and I went to bed for the night. *That's what I really need*, I thought. A full night's sleep would set me right—wouldn't it?

5

An Uncomfortable Flight

The inevitable is, inevitably, inevitable.
—William F. Buckley

April 25, 2024, Thursday

My plan of waking up without a fever and with a feeling of general strength didn't happen. I felt as bad Thursday morning as I had the night before—and as I slid out of bed, I suddenly noticed two irritating small dots, one on my right ankle and the other on my upper left thigh. My first thought was that maybe I had been bitten by something while in bed; Hawaii is fortunate not to have many pesky insects, but who could say a spider hadn't visited us at night?

When I mentioned the bug bites to Peggy, she said it was odd that she hadn't been eaten up by them, since she was typically the one who got bitten, not me. Bugs seemed to be out of the equation. As I inspected my foot more closely, I realized the dots looked a bit more like puncture wounds, and there wasn't a welt like you'd expect with a bite or sting. If I'd stepped on a thumbtack, I would have expected my skin to look the same way.

I still hadn't told her about getting zapped during Tuesday's swim because by now, I'd forgotten it happened—and since she didn't know about the jellyfish sting, there was no reason for her to connect the dots, figuratively or literally. As Sherlock Holmes once said, "The world is full of obvious things which nobody by any chance ever observes." Looking back, that feels painfully true. My withholding wasn't some premeditated attempt to sabotage the solving of a mystery; I was unwittingly adding to the high-stakes suspense. Once I was stung, my mind, body, and—surprisingly—my memory were already beginning to fail.

I went about my usual morning routine as best I could and noticed I was hobbling a bit. My foot with the puncture wounds was tender and felt a bit numb the more I walked on it. When I mentioned this new development to Peggy, her solution was to give me ibuprofen to reduce the swelling and to elevate and ice my foot. I could tell that none of this was adding up for her. "Do you want to stay and wait this out and depart the island Sunday?" she asked.

That was a smart suggestion—dealing with travel and time changes is enough to discourage even a healthy traveler, and I would have stayed if I'd thought I was overly contagious or had a viral infection. To rule that out, Peggy had even given me a COVID test the night before that came up negative. There was no good reason not to travel, so when she asked me if I wanted to delay our upcoming flight, I felt a resolution welling up inside me.

"No, let's stick with the schedule," I replied. "San Francisco is a good spot to see a doctor if I need one."

This was one of those silent crossroads, a single decision that could have life-changing consequences. I didn't know it at the time, but my insistence on keeping to the schedule saved my life.

Peggy insisted that I retake my temperature—100.1°F—which hadn't changed much from the day before. I congratulated myself for being consistent, and after I'd iced my foot for twenty minutes or so, I continued to get ready for the day. Our flight was scheduled to depart at 1:00 p.m., and the airport was only ten minutes away from our house. Peggy had plenty of time for her regular morning workout, and we were able to take care of a few last-minute things to wrap up our long stay.

As we made our rounds that morning, the aching in my foot steadily increased, slowly creeping up into my leg. It felt like I had been sitting with my legs crossed for too long, and my right leg had fallen asleep. That deep tingling numbness came and went as we went about our morning. Sometimes I'd bump my leg against the edge of a chair or something else sturdy and stationary and it felt like an old motorcycle had been kickstarted. Every time I'd brush my right leg against something, the numbness would disappear for a few seconds, offering a moment of relief.

There came a point in our morning outing when Peggy and I were hanging out with a friend and in the middle of the conversation, I needed everything to stop. That was highly unusual for me—I'm a social person, and I'd long ago mastered the art of slipping out of a conversation when I needed to. But this wasn't about being tired of the person. I felt an urgent need for a full stop. I turned to Peggy and expressed my feelings the only way I knew how: "I can't stay here any longer. Can we leave?"

The question was as far out of left field for me to say as it was for her to hear. By that point, she was flummoxed by my lingering symptoms and behavior. She'd caught sight of me nursing my leg, too. Peggy, always perceptive, had been watching me more closely than I realized. She didn't say anything right away, but I could tell her mind was racing to connect the dots—I, too, was struggling to do so. I couldn't find the words to explain what was happening inside me, but we silently came to the same conclusion: We needed to get me off the island and back to the mainland.

On our way back to the house, I knew Peggy was still trying to work everything out. Then, out of nowhere, she said, "Bees. Maybe it was your bees."

Beekeeping was one of my hobbies, and we kept a hive in the side yard, but I hadn't been out to check on my little pollinators all week. Unless a few bees had hunted me down in the house, I doubted it was them.

The bee theory ended with us returning to the house to finish packing. That wasn't much of a chore. We kept clothes in Hawaii and only needed small travel bags of essentials for our next warm-weather destination. Still, packing was difficult for me. Walking was irritating my right foot, and it felt like I was losing more sensation there as time went on. Every step was uncomfortable, but the persistent throbbing is what was getting to me. I couldn't understand why the quality of my ache wasn't lessening with Tylenol.

The plane ride is where my memory starts getting shaky, but I know the flight went without a hitch. There weren't many people on the plane, so luckily, I was able to stretch out—that was a bonus, but it didn't help as much as I thought it would. When we got to altitude, my foot started swelling even more. I shifted. I turned. But I couldn't get comfortable. Eventually, I took my shoes off. That gave me some blessed relief for a while, but by now, the skin on my right foot felt taut and slick, like it was covered in a boil. I kept downing Advil and Tylenol throughout the flight and started icing my foot again.

My memory has tried to convince me that I kept going to sleep and waking up, but that probably wasn't the case—brain fog was likely setting in. My focus kept waxing and waning to the point that I didn't understand why Peggy announced she was looking up doctors and hospitals in San Francisco. It sounded vaguely reasonable, but I couldn't quite connect the dots.

During the flight, Peggy had made contact and sent an image to our primary doctor in Idaho, Dr. Tom Archie. He said that I likely had a rapid progression of cellulitis from bug bites, which could cause a fever and would require antibiotics. *My best advice is that John should see somebody in an ER after landing*, he replied in a text exchange.

Five hours later, the airplane skidded to a halt on the runway and taxied to our departure point. I got off the aircraft and followed Peggy like a puppy to the Uber that was waiting for us. Thinking ahead, Peggy called the hotel from the car. Putting aside Dr. Archie's advice for a moment, she asked the hotel concierge if they could refer us to an on-call doctor who might see me after 10:00 p.m.—she was concerned that the nearest ER was outdated and wouldn't be fully equipped. We were unaware that California Pacific Medical Center had recently completed a new hospital location nearby, and of course, neither of us truly understood how serious my condition was. If we had, we wouldn't have hesitated to follow Dr. Archie's recommendation.

"I don't know of anyone who has used this particular service, but there's an on-call doctor, Dr. Savage, who has been recommended from time to time," the hotel concierge replied. "We can call and let him know you're coming. Would you like me to do that for you?"

Peggy immediately agreed, and the front desk staff went into action. One of them called Dr. Savage, another arranged for a cab to take us there, and another instructed the bellhop to carry our luggage to our room. We were in a cab within minutes.

Getting a one-on-one with a doctor after the dinner hour was enough of a miracle that we didn't stop to think why a doctor who wasn't on staff in a hospital would agree to see a patient after 10:00 p.m. Had we come across his Yelp reviews, we likely would have gone somewhere else:

If you told me he had done a bump of coke before finally starting my appointment, I would absolutely believe you. He was extremely high energy, talking a mile-a-minute and at one point, literally jumping up and down.

The taxi driver stopped the car and told us we had arrived. We paid the cabbie, and he didn't stick around to see if we got in the building. Even in my diminished state, I could tell we weren't in the best part of downtown San Francisco. *Once we get in the building, we'll be okay*, I thought as Peggy pulled on the front door.

It was locked.

She knocked on the glass door, but there was no immediate response. She glanced over at me with frustration and concern, then tried again, louder this time. She pulled out her phone to call Dr. Savage, telling him we were locked out downstairs. After five long minutes passed, a security guard unlocked the door and opened it only enough to stick his nose through.

"Dr. Savage, we're here to see Dr. Savage," Peggy said with urgency.

Recognition lit up the guard's face as he opened the door fully and ushered us inside. In that neighborhood, I wouldn't have been surprised if all sorts of people wanted to loiter in the lobby. I probably would have barricaded myself inside, too, if I had been the one on the night shift here.

After passing through the entrance, the guard pointed us to the elevator and told us which floor we needed. I could feel Peggy's hand squeezing my arm tightly as we stepped into the elevator. The tension in her body was palpable as the numbers on display beeped with each floor we passed.

When we located Dr. Savage's office, he was already deeply engrossed in a conversation with another patient. More accurately, Dr. Savage was in the middle of a monologue—his hands gestured wildly, his voice rapid and upbeat, as if he were giving a TED Talk rather than attending to someone's medical concerns.

Peggy cleared her throat loudly, trying to get his assistant's attention, but she barely glanced in our direction. Minutes ticked by as Dr. Savage continued his energetic ramblings and his assistant ignored that we were impatiently waiting just a few feet away. Peggy could tell my discomfort had intensified as I sat down in one of the stiff chairs, wondering if we'd ever be acknowledged.

"My husband is in agony and needs to be seen now," she said as sternly as her exhausted body could muster. The doctor eventually wrapped up his conversation and motioned for us to come back to the exam room. He asked me what had happened over the last few days while he did the initial assessment. I info-dumped, telling Dr. Savage everything I could remember from the last forty-eight hours or so—well, almost everything. In my delirium, I once again didn't see a connection between the jellyfish sting and the swelling, so it wasn't brought up.

Dr. Savage didn't give much of a diagnosis, but he did select a course of treatment. "I'm going to give you some antibiotics, pain medicine, and Ambien to help you sleep." I nodded, and he gave me a week's worth of oral antibiotics. "Call me if you need anything else," he said. Then, he motioned for me to turn around so he could give me a shot on my backside. The shot was three different formulas in the same syringe: an antibiotic, lidocaine, and something else. Peggy was distraught with what he was doing but trusted him—he was, after all, a doctor.

"What do we do if it gets worse?" I asked on our way out the door.

"Here's my card," he offered to Peggy. "You call me."

On the ride back to the hotel, my pain eased up slightly. It went from hammer and tongs striking at my bones to extreme discomfort. That was a win. I looked over at Peggy and wished Dr. Savage had given her something to help her calm down. She looked exhausted enough to not even be able to sleep once we got back to the room, though thankfully, that wasn't the case. Peggy placed the doctor's business card on my bedside table and drifted off almost as soon as we got settled, though I suspected she wouldn't be asleep for more than half an hour.

It was a different story for me. Once again, I could not find a comfortable position. I don't know if I ever went to sleep or was caught in that foggy stage before dreamland, but at some point, something forced me fully awake. The pain in my foot was back—full throttle. I'd had enough. I grabbed my phone and found Dr. Savage's card. My fingers were slightly unsteady as I tapped the number, barely registering that it was just after midnight. I must've punched in the number correctly because, within seconds, Dr. Savage picked up.

"Dr. Savage, this is John. I was just in. I'm feeling worse. What should I do?"

Peggy sat straight up when I started talking. She was looking expectantly at me, already grabbing for her clothes.

"Go straight to the California Pacific Medical Center ER. It's not far from your hotel, and they've got a good emergency department."

That was all I needed to hear.

Peggy went into crisis mode and got dressed faster than I think she ever had in her life. I was sitting on the bed's edge like a zombie, and I heard her say, "John—John! You've got to get dressed. We're going to get you to the ER."

At nearly 1:00 a.m., it would have been easier to dress a toddler. I put on my pants and belt, which, given the circumstances, was an accomplishment. Real shoes were out of the question with my lethargic behavior and unbearable foot pain, so I gently slid my feet into the hotel slippers.

Downstairs, Peggy loaded me into an Uber, the last thing I would remember clearly for the next three days.

6

Roots in San Francisco

As a parent, it's my priority to help you into Heaven, not Harvard.

—Anonymous

In the movies, this would likely be the point where the main character would look back on his life. In my case, there would be a montage of all my life events leading me to the precipice of my brain failing to retain memories as Peggy anxiously gripped my hand in the back of the Uber, all with a celebrity voiceover describing each of the major events of my life in pithy detail until we arrived at the ER. I was deprived of my flashback moment, because I was completely out of it. You could have told me Martians just invaded, and I wouldn't have known any better.

Strangely, though, when I try to recall our arrival at the ER, searching my mind for what happened next, I don't go forward. I go backward. My thoughts drift to the sixty years that led me to that moment, as if my brain, scrambling to ground itself, starts reaching for the earliest threads of my identity. It makes sense, I suppose. I entered the world on October 25, 1963, at Children's Hospital in San Francisco—not far from where I now felt perilously close to exiting it.

Much of whatever success I've had in life began with the good fortune of being born the second son of Bruce Drown Baker and Barbara Breyer Baker, parents who observed the differences between their three sons and ultimately understood how to calmly guide each one in their own respective directions. They understood the value of adventure and the great outdoors, providing us opportunities to build our self-esteem as Cub Scouts, on after school sports teams, and through summers of backpacking and adventure.

My father had his own quiet strength, shaped in part by his service in the Navy during the Cold War, about fourteen years after the end of World War II. He had just graduated from UC Berkeley—where he'd met my mother—when he enlisted, deploying only a few months later. They were engaged at the time and got married soon after at St. John's Episcopal Church in Ross, California, to ensure that they could stay together during his service. It was a quiet, heartfelt decision rooted in love and a shared sense of duty.

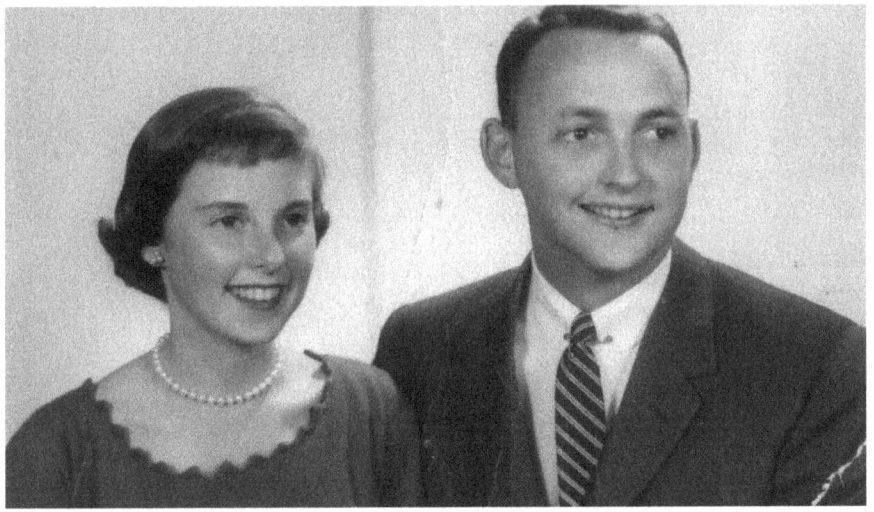

My parents, Bruce and Barbara Baker, 1959

His assignment took them to Adak Island, part of Alaska's remote Aleutian chain a thousand miles from the mainland. My mother followed him there, working in the supply center and post office while he served as a communications officer. Much of his time was spent inside an isolated bunker, typing encrypted messages on a machine designed to protect national secrets. It was isolated, cold, and far from the world they knew—but they were together. I've always admired the quiet courage it must have taken to build their marriage in the early days under such conditions.

When they returned to San Francisco, they began the next chapter of their life together. My father started a career in insurance, eventually partnering with Don Sweet in 1975 to create Sweet & Baker Insurance. The business grew steadily, with a loyal Bay Area clientele, and ultimately sold to Hubb Insurance around the time my dad retired in 2017.

In those early years, my mom worked in the business, too, managing the bookkeeping while raising three energetic boys. She was the steady hand behind the scenes, loyal, resilient, and unwavering in her support for my father and the life they were building. Their bond was steady and unspoken, the kind of partnership that didn't need to announce itself in order to be deeply felt. Together, they built a stable life, a comfortable home, and the foundation of a family that would grow out of their lasting union.

Our first home was at 279 28th Avenue, between California and Lake Streets. We were a solidly middle-class family living on the fringes of a neighborhood called Sea Cliff, a scenic enclave known for its sweeping views of the bridge and its proximity to Baker Beach—of no relation, that I'm aware of.

When I was almost four, and with my soon-to-be-brother Chris on his way, we moved across the alley to 274 29th Avenue, into a bigger house with space for our growing family. Over the

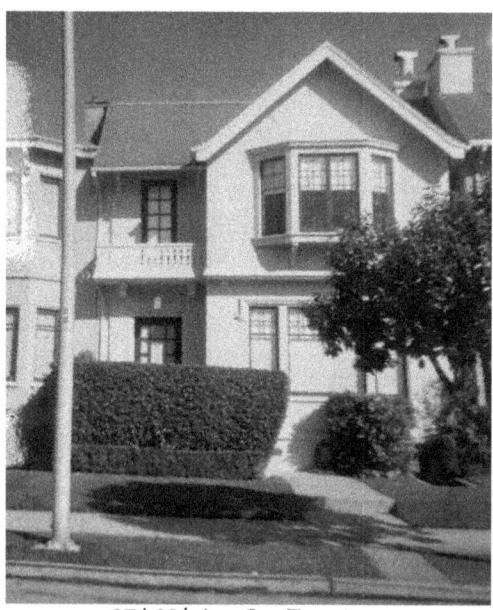

274 29th Ave, San Francisco, the home where I spent most of my childhood

years, my mom has said the move may have been what triggered her labor with my younger brother—I remember helping to carry a few small items from the old house to the new one, barely understanding what it all meant. The new place had lots of small rooms and a long, narrow garage that could hold three cars, end to end. It was comfortable, and it was home.

Heart of the Journey

The best part was living on a street filled with young families, where all the kids ran in a pack and grew up together. Life was simpler back then: the newspaper was delivered to our doorstep, fresh milk arrived courtesy of the milkman, and our cloth diapers were taken away for washing—and all this commerce happened without the benefits of DoorDash or Uber. I grew up in an analog age of needing to memorize phone numbers, with carbon paper as our version of copy/paste.

In the back of the house, just outside the basement, was the small yard I loved spending time in after finishing any chores and homework—and just outside our backyard was "the alley," a dead-end street where all the neighborhood kids gathered to play dodgeball, kickball, basketball, and hide-and-seek. It was a place where we could dream big dreams, but also where we learned to work together, solve problems, and be socially and physically active; perhaps it was what sparked my desires for adventure and constant activity later in life.

The alley provided its lessons, but the bulk of my memories and early life lessons came from inside my childhood house, where every room carried its own story. In the center of the kitchen sat an island table, small and unassuming but bursting with versatility. It was one of those old-fashioned tables on small metal casters with wooden sides that could fold out from underneath so that you could expand its surface as needed.

The kitchen table was a landing place for homework papers, mail, notes, and groceries. It witnessed our messes, joys, jumbled belongings, and scattered thoughts, always providing a sense of steadiness amidst any chaos. In many ways, it was the heart of our home, a silent witness to the ebb and flow of family life.

Also in that kitchen, on the side counter, was a little bowl filled with nickels for the city bus that stopped half a block from our house. If you grabbed a couple nickels as you headed out the door, you could catch it and ride the bus to school or wherever you wanted to go. It symbolized the start of countless journeys and became a lifeline of sorts, though not because we wanted to get away from home. We viewed it as an easy way to access other neighborhoods and visit our friends. While the kitchen was the launch pad for our daily routines, that little bowl of nickels was the currency.

The kitchen opened into a narrow hallway that led toward the front of the house. A Persian carpet covered the hardwood floor, which my mother loved, and an ornate grandfather clock added a touch of elegance to the otherwise utilitarian space. Passed down from my grandparents, it stood tall in the middle of the staircase as a constant reminder of passing time. The hands on the clock face moved ever so slowly, no matter how much I wanted them to speed up at times. You had to wind the clock by hand, and its chime was a part of the background music of our lives. It was romantic, in a way, but also a little haunting. The tick-tocks and chimes of the clock always made me think the clock knew more about our family than we did.

Beyond the clock, you'd reach a modest set of carpeted stairs with a right turn to another landing, continuing up another seven or eight steps to the second floor. At the top, the staircase opened into a square landing, a common area connecting all the bedrooms and our shared bathroom. In my late teenage years, when I would come home late on weekends, I'd hug the far left side of the staircase, careful to avoid the squeaky steps, fooling myself into thinking my mother hadn't heard me slip in.

On the second floor and off to the right was my parents' room, a space I rarely ventured into except to watch the evening news with Walter Cronkite or game shows like *The Price Is Right*—or to see what Christmas presents were hiding on the top shelf of my mother's closet during the holidays after sneaking in when nobody was home.

My younger brother Chris had a room adjacent to mine, with two other doors off the hall—one leading into our shared bathroom and the other into a small linen closet. My older brother Wayne's room was at the back of the house, though it felt more like a sun porch. It didn't retain heat very well with single-paned glass windows on two sides, but for some reason, he liked it that way. To get to his room, you had to walk through mine or take a parallel path through Chris's room.

My room was simple and all mine. Its walls were covered in a light blue wallpaper that had a fine checkered pattern, terminating at a small picture molding. Above that, a section of white wall ran up to the ceiling. In the middle of the ceiling was a single light fixture shaped like a lantern and controlled by a dimmer switch on the wall.

Centered in my room against the wall was a single bed with a wooden headboard, a piece of furniture that felt sturdy and old, much like the house itself. To the left of the bed was my study desk and to the right, a dresser. Later, I inherited a large mahogany dresser from my grandfather, replacing the small four-drawer bureau that held my clothes for so many years.

My desk was where I spent countless hours trying to study, dreaming of more productive activities like being with friends and going on adventures. The walls were thin and nearby homes were stacked side-by-side, so I was often distracted by the next-door neighbors' elevated voices or their barking dachshund named Mighty Mite.

A welcoming distraction usually came in the early evenings, when my neighbor, Renee Goddard, would knock on the sheet metal drainpipe that was just outside the right of my window and flanked the neighbor's property, where Renee lived. She and I grew closer around the age of fourteen, when we realized we shared so many mutual friends. We never went to the same schools—in fact, our schools were semi-rivals—but our window talks allowed us to catch up on all the gossip. *Does Greg still like Francesca? I can't believe Jenny and Griff are still together! Who are you inviting to the prom?* Even though our lives are different and we live far apart, Renee has been a constant in my life. It has been, by far, the longest-lasting friendship either of us has ever had.

***

Despite the fond memories, my room wasn't always a place of comfort. Studying was never easy for me—in fact, it was often deeply frustrating. I struggled in school, constantly feeling behind and as though I needed twice the time just to keep up. Each afternoon, I felt confined in the quiet of my room until the day's homework was finished, only to be distracted by the other neighboring kids playing in the alley. I spent long hours at that desk—often pleading for help, which my mother selflessly and patiently provided—as I tried to grasp concepts that always seemed just out of reach.

I attended Town School for Boys from 1970 to 1976, repeating first grade because I was young for my class and my reading skills needed work.

My mother later realized I had dyslexia, although I was never officially diagnosed. For me, being dyslexic felt like my brain processed words and letters differently, making reading and writing a constant puzzle to solve, since words could seem to blur or flip (which is often still frustrating). The malady also wasn't something that most teachers knew about in the early 1970s. Everyone knew I was smart, so they assumed I must be lazy, or that I didn't care about my schoolwork. It was why my mother kept me in my room to do my homework. She believed I just needed to focus, and quiet time seemed like the obvious solution. Over time, I learned to navigate dyslexia with patience and creative strategies. Thankfully, I never let it define me.

Concentrating on my studies felt a little easier knowing I had support, but the afternoons weren't any easier with my older brother Wayne right next door. He was always quick to remind me when I was being too loud or did the slightest thing that annoyed him. In his eyes, I'm sure I was the needy younger brother taking all the attention. Still, I respected his independence and sharp wit, even when we clashed. It wasn't until much later in life—over family dinners and phone calls—that we found real common ground. These days, our conversations are heartfelt and filled with mutual respect, something I'm grateful for.

Chris, on the other hand, was just a baby when we moved into the house. We were four years apart, and in those early years, I didn't pay much attention to him. At the time, he was the same needy little brother to me that I was to Wayne. But as we got older, I began to see him differently. By the time I was in high school, we developed a close bond that made up for the distance we'd felt in those early years. Today, I consider him not just a brother but one of my closest friends. He'll often check in with a call or a text, asking for older brother advice—which I gladly provide, even if he doesn't take it.

Heart of the Journey

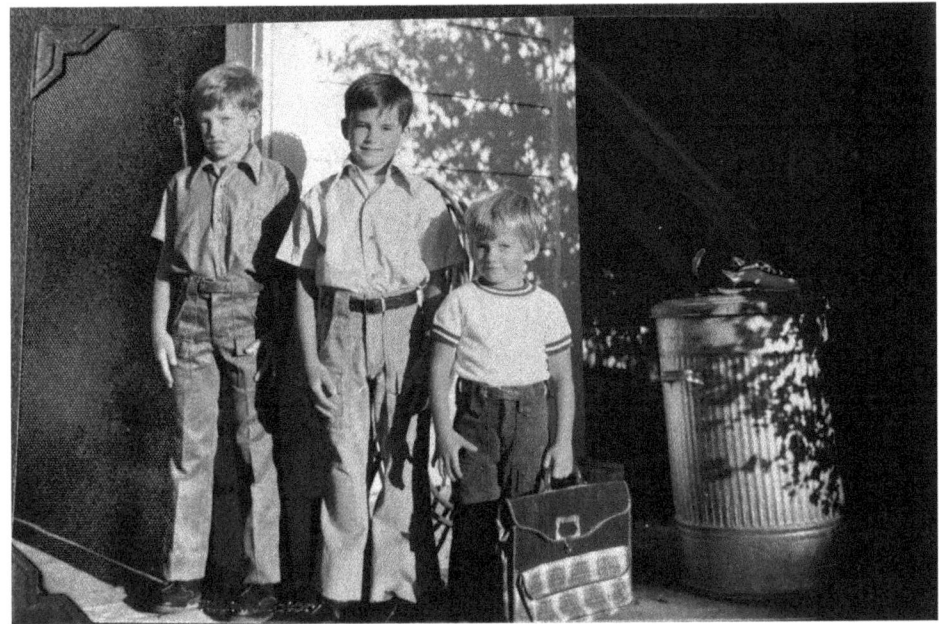

First day of school with brothers Wayne and Chris, 1972

***

My life's most lasting lessons haven't been confined to four walls. As much as my family and our home on 29th Avenue shaped the man I would become, so too did the city of San Francisco, with its vibrant neighborhoods and affluent circles.

Though our home offered all the familiar comforts, it felt removed from the heart of the city, where our schools were located along with many of my closest friends. We weren't exactly in the thick of Haight-Ashbury's psychedelic pulse, either, yet the spirit of the late 1960s lingered in the air. The hippie influence clung to San Francisco like a Grateful Dead song—it was as if "Terrapin Station" had been playing in the background of my youth—but our home stood in quiet contrast to that countercultural energy.

The house itself held a quiet duality. And yet, with my mother's patient and unwavering support throughout my grammar school years, it slowly became a place of growth—a space where, without realizing it, I began to build confidence in other ways. I found myself more willing to try new things, to step outside my comfort zone, and to keep moving forward.

I remember the stairs that always announced my arrival with a creak. I remember studying beside the heat vent, waiting for the forced-air unit two floors below to kick back on. I remember the loud hum of the nearby Muni bus as it came to a stop just an earshot away. I remember the rumbling of the garage door opening as my father came home from work, and the distant call of foghorns coming over the Golden Gate Bridge.

In its own way, the house became a quiet companion to my early story. I suppose that's what ultimately makes a house a home—not just the people who live in it, but how it holds the memories of both our struggles and our joy.

7

Golden Days

*It's not what we have in our life,
but who we have in our life that matters.*

—Anonymous

As I grew older, life expanded beyond our block and the alley, beyond those early friendships. In sixth grade, I transferred from Town School to Stuart Hall, where the teachers gave me the extra attention I needed. They saw a spark in me, something worth nurturing, and with their support, I managed to finish each year with decent grades. Around that same time, I was beginning to navigate the complexities of relationships, particularly with girls. Robin Hauser was my first girlfriend. Our relationship was innocent—holding hands, talking on the phone, and being paired up at dancing school—but at the time, it felt monumental.

It's funny to think back on those moments now. My younger brother, even at such a young age, was acquainted with Robin's younger sister. I'd get on the phone with Robin, and after we talked for a moment, I'd hand the phone to Chris as Robin handed her phone to her sister. For a few short moments we'd go on trading the receiver back and forth until one of our mothers said "enough." If an important call were to come in, you didn't want to have them get the busy signal.

It wasn't until much later that I realized how different my path might have been if I'd had access to the kinds of resources available to kids today—

more widespread recognition of learning differences and regular tutoring support. I had some professional help here and there, but mostly, it was my mother who stepped in and did her best to help me navigate the maze of academics.

All the while, my parents' lives were tightly bound by the demands of running a small business and raising a family. Yet despite the pressures, they instilled in us not only a strong work ethic but a deep love for the outdoors, something my father had embraced as a boy during backpacking trips with the Sierra Club. There was nothing extravagant about it, just simple, meaningful moments of connection with nature. When my father had a break from work or family demands, he spent it doing what he loved most: fly-fishing. He was a devoted angler, with a keen eye, strong casting skills, and above all, patience.

Some of my most vivid memories of those adolescent and early teenage years were our trips to the High Sierras, where my father learned to fly-fish with his father. He always found the most pristine alpine lakes to pursue his passion. His parents, Virginia and Harry Baker (we called them Nana and Papa), loved the outdoors as well and carried on a tradition of taking us on annual outings to either a dude ranch or the Mackenzie River. On the Mackenzie, we would float in dory boats, consuming whatever trout we caught at the fish fry that day on the riverbank—it was amazing how a stick of butter could make those fish taste so good. Nana even used to eat the fisheyes, calling them a delicacy.

During my early school years, weekends were often spent in Marin County, either at the home of my maternal grandparents, Stan and Terry Breyer, or at Paul Dailey's Swim and Tennis Club. My father, always looking for weekend adventures, often motivated me to ride the seventeen miles across the Golden Gate Bridge to Mill Valley on my bike to the racket club. I still remember the exhilaration of those rides, cresting the Camino Alto grade, with him pointing out Bill Graham's house (the first promoter of the Grateful Dead) as we flew down the back roads into Larkspur. We'd all finish the day playing tennis, swimming, or just diving into the pool. Of course, the Buick family wagon was the preferred ride back over the bridge to our home in the city.

Besides babysitting in my early teens, my first real job and taste of responsibility was stringing rackets and helping run the small tennis shop at Paul Dailey's when the pro was out giving lessons. The recognition and achievement that came with working felt good, even at such a young age. It set me apart from the other kids in some ways, gave me confidence, and, perhaps, laid the foundation for the work ethic that would carry me through the years to come.

There were also moments of pure exhilaration, like running the Bay to Breakers, San Francisco's iconic footrace known for its quirky, festive atmosphere. Race participants often wore elaborate costumes—or nothing at all. The race spans twelve kilometers, starting near the Embarcadero by the Bay and finishing at the Great Highway and Ocean Beach.

Running the Bay to Breakers became another Baker family tradition. It wasn't just a running race. The Bay to Breakers was a rite of passage, a celebration of life wrapped in an athletic achievement. When we finished the race near Playland at Ocean Beach, the fog would be rolling in, but our weary bodies would still be energized from the cold and the thrill of accomplishing the run.

Understandably, many of my friends didn't see the point of me running all the way across the city just for the sport of it. But running, as well as skiing, prepared me to chart my own athletic path as I got older.

Most winter weekends of my childhood, we'd head up to the Sierra Mountains for the sheer exhilaration of it. My parents strapped skis on me when I was just four years old. Back then, kids could ski all day for free at many of the resorts around Lake Tahoe.

I was so obsessed with skiing that I had a ridiculous poster in my bedroom that read SKI NEBRASKA. It showed a guy in full ski gear trying to pole through a field of dead corn stalks. It made me smile every time I saw it—because when I'd been off the slopes too long, even a cornfield started to look skiable.

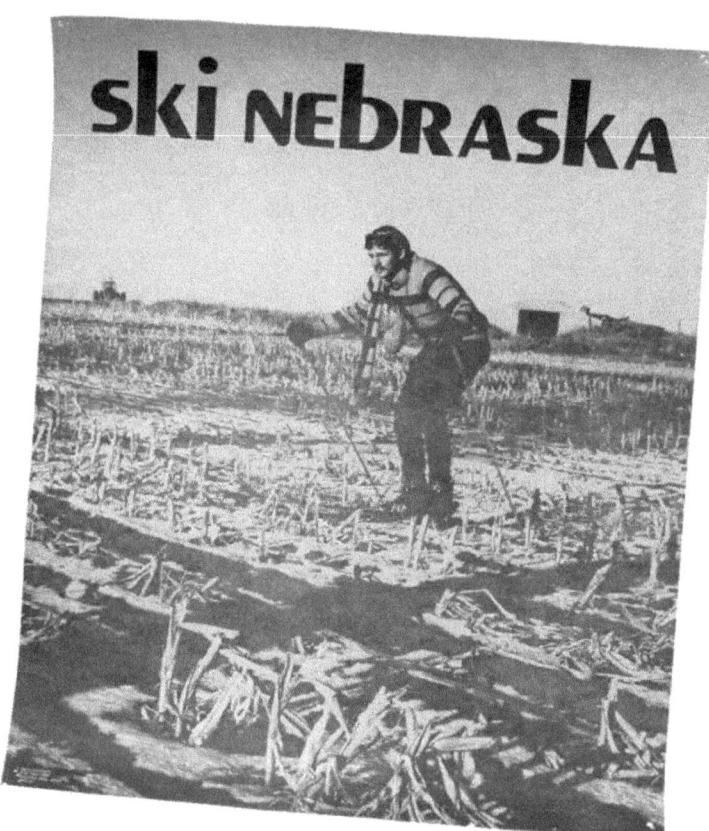

The *Ski Nebraska* poster that hung in my room

8

Learning My Own Way

Luck is when opportunity meets preparation.
—Anonymous

As a calculating numbers guy, it's important that I try to understand the unseen universe. That realm lies somewhere between quantum physics and magic, where unseen forces direct our lives in specific paths. I know there must be something akin to fate or luck, because my life is a testament to either being at the right place at the right time or having the right people cross my path when I needed them most. Whether destiny or pure chance, I've learned to recognize those invisible forces that seem to guide me toward unexpected opportunities and outcomes.

I also think that whatever mojo kicks us around this life depends on how an individual reacts to those opportunities. Life is a cascading event where one experience prepares us for something else. That something else could be getting your dream job, surviving a crisis, or meeting that certain someone. As I look back on the adventures of my youth, I see a straight line through all those things.

While the days spent with friends were marked by carefree fun, our family vacations in my teens took us on journeys that would subtly shape my drive and determination. We often ventured to Lake Tahoe, a place that became synonymous with exploration and, as I grew older, hard work. Summers were spent adventuring through the pristine wilderness, and my father was always eager to tackle a new challenge. One of our most memorable adventures in Tahoe was cycling from Squaw Valley to Donner Summit. As I pushed myself up old Highway 40, my legs burned from the climb. I felt that familiar mix of exhaustion and triumph—a theme that would follow me throughout my life.

My father had an affinity for the dramatic (in the physical sense), for experiences that pushed the boundaries of comfort. He rode in the Davis Double Century, a grueling, 200-mile ride completed in a single day under the scorching heat of Sacramento. Another time, he rode his bicycle with a pal from San Diego to the tip of Baja, seeking safe shelter in the evenings to get some rest. One weekend when I was fifteen, we boxed up our road bikes and took a Greyhound bus north to Eureka, California. We rode three hundred miles back to San Francisco, through the towering redwoods along the coast. The rain and wind made the two-day ride punishing. In such situations, you don't know whether to hate the person who suggested the trip or love them more for creating the memory. I'm sure there was a bit of both—especially as the icy rain relentlessly pelted my face.

The weather wasn't the only hazard. While riding behind my father, I relied on a small, helmet-mounted rearview mirror to warn him of massive logging trucks barreling toward us from behind. The eighteen-wheelers forced us to the side of the road every time they approached. Was it dangerous? Yes, it was. Did my father and I become more connected by the end of the trip? Of course we did.

I recall trailing behind, exhausted, and yelling, "Hey, Dad, are we almost there?" with slight impatience as a large logging truck overtook us without warning, the noise almost blocking out his words.

"Yes, son, we're getting closer," he responded, knowing that offering a vague response was all he could do. I recall feeling let down that he didn't know exactly how long in minutes or even seconds. It was one of the early times in my life I had to put my head down and dig deep, as I wasn't getting to the finish line any other way but through grit and determination. Aside from the trauma bonding, I had the chance to share an unforgettable adventure with him, though I was most relieved to greet my mother at the Golden Gate finish.

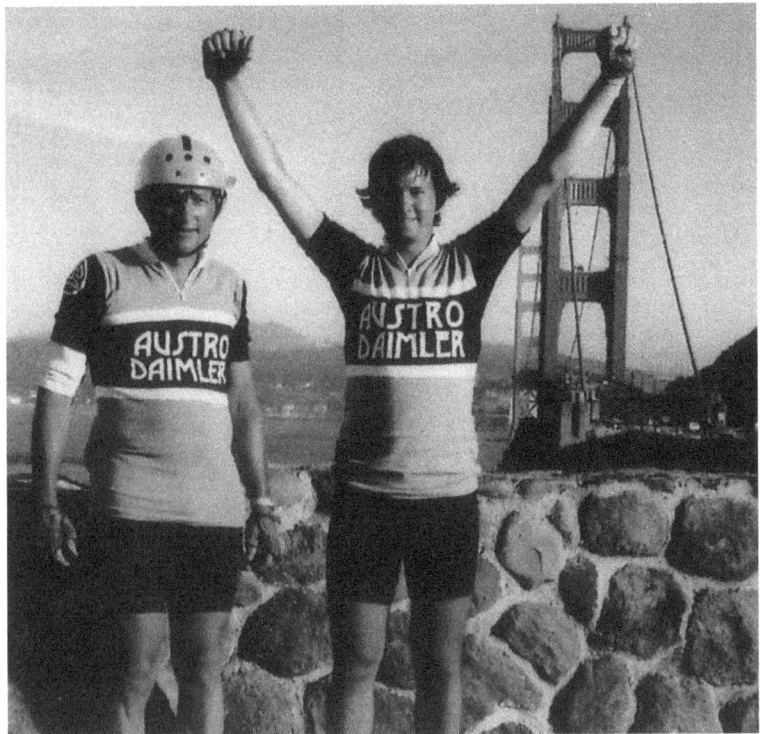

Early athletic feats with my father

Not all my summers were spent on fun and adventures; more often than not, they were spent working. Little did I know that my winding path to a fulfilling career would begin during my high school summers of 1978 to 1982. My folks bought a small house in Squaw Valley, which is now known as Palisades Tahoe, my freshman year in high school, sharing it with the Kirkpatrick family of six. A second home would be a more precise term. I was there all four summers during my high school years, taking on various jobs in Squaw Valley and the towns that surround Lake Tahoe.

As a teenager, I was personable and not too shy when speaking with adults—and if you can hold your own in a conversation with adults, jobs tend to come more easily. I quickly became skilled with the cash register at every job I had. There's something invaluable about handling tangible money at a young age—it's an experience that's rare for kids today. My son Wilson once famously asked, "Why do I need to learn to count change when you can just use a credit card?"

My first job during freshman summer of high school was flipping Quarter Pounders at McDonald's in Tahoe City. After a month of adhering to Mickey D's strict protocols, I was offered to manage Big Red's Chicken & Spaghetti takeout down the street from McDonald's for the rest of the summer. Fast food wasn't exactly my dream job, so I moved on to something more exciting the following summer: Mumbo's Mountain Shop. This small, family-run outdoor retailer sold a wide variety of gear for mountain enthusiasts. I did well at Mumbo's, with the exception of my grave error of using a box cutter to open new inventory. There I was, happily slicing through box after box, when I realized I was cutting into the expensive rafts packaged inside. I discovered just how costly a small mistake could be, both financially and personally. Thankfully, I didn't suffer any consequences, although I'm sure the shop lost money due to my mistake. Through every misstep, I grew more resilient and more determined.

The tension between struggle and success shaped these formative years. Whether it was grappling with dyslexia in the classroom or pushing myself in other work areas, I learned that perseverance was my greatest asset.

***

I wasn't the top athlete in school, but I was good enough. I excelled early on in baseball, soccer, tennis, and skiing, giving me a sense of purpose and, if I'm honest, a bit of swagger. The girls noticed, and so did I. High school brought new connections and challenges and solidified some of my closest relationships, including one with an inspiring human named Beau Giannini. His family home embodied a wider world for me—a constant whirlwind of activity with four siblings and friends constantly coming and going. I spent countless hours there, including weekend overnights, relishing the revolving door energy that starkly contrasted the quieter rhythm of life at home.

Beau has remained one of my best friends to this day, as we shared experiences that are still seared into our memories. What makes our friendship endure is its simplicity. There are no hidden agendas, no envy, no jealousy—just transparency. We've gone years without seeing each other only to pick up exactly where we left off. Even our daughters have forged their own friendship in New York, joining the same book club and exploring restaurants together, a second generation of connection that neither of us forced, but both of us cherish.

I often found my connections with motivated, positive people, and Stephano Bini (*yes, another Italian!*) was also a partner in crime back then. Beau and I had a grand adventure visiting him and his extended family in their hometown of Arezzo, Italy. Stephano's father was an inspiring architect, which may have further influenced my decision later on to choose architecture as my major in college.

In my junior year at Lick-Wilmerding High School in San Francisco, I took a drafting class and was introduced further into the world of architecture. I became fascinated with designing and building. At home, I'd always taken on minor household maintenance projects, to my mother's delight. There was something about that kind of work that just made sense to me. I could look at whatever needed to be fixed, and somehow, from the basics I'd learned, I knew how to make the problem disappear. So that junior summer, when I returned to Lake Tahoe, I'd had enough of working in fast food or shops. Instead, I applied to work for a contractor as a general laborer on a home being built in Alpine Meadows.

I didn't have a car then, so I made the roundtrip from Squaw to the Alpine jobsite every day on my bike. Imagine biking five miles along the river and up the mountain road just to start a manual labor job. I remember one of my duties on that beautiful hillside home was carrying five-gallon buckets of dirt and rocks along wooden planks to backfill concrete retaining walls. I had learned a little about mythology in school, and at first, carrying thousands of heavy five-gallon buckets made me feel like Sisyphus. He was a cunning king, condemned by the gods to an eternal punishment of rolling a boulder up a hill. Once the boulder neared the top of the hill, it would roll back down again to its base. Day after day, Sisyphus was doomed never to see his work accomplish anything.

But after a week or so, I forgot about Sisyphus. I started to see what I and the other workers were accomplishing. Typically, where there were once land, rocks, and trees, the shape of a house would emerge. This particular home, however, was thoughtfully designed around some of the natural features of the property, such as the large boulder formations. The architecture embraced the formations, incorporating them into the finished design. In fact, the saying "the boulders were there first" really resonated with me. Everyone on the job contributed to the home being built—even me, a dyslexic, shiny-faced teenager. That was a feeling of accomplishment I would never have gotten at the Golden Arches or Big Red's Chicken & Spaghetti. It wasn't like those customers called back after their meal, telling you how the food changed their lives. But with a home, I was helping to build a place where families grew and made memories. I never wanted to return to food service or retail again, even though ringing that cash register sure felt satisfying.

The following summer, after graduating from high school, my friend Griff Towle and I went rogue. We operated as independent contractors, staining houses together. Griff and I were young, ambitious, and determined to make our mark. Every morning, we'd load up Griff's primer grey BMW 2002, an old but undeniably cool icon of its time, with linseed oil and ladders. Linseed oil was the best wood finish for the high mountain area—it penetrated deep into the wood, providing a natural, durable finish that protected the houses from the harsh elements. It was our secret weapon, giving every house we worked on a fresh coat that made it look new again. That's the attention to detail ruining a dozen rubber rafts teaches you.

Griff and I felt the pressure of upcoming college that summer. My parents were paying generously for four years of school; however, I wasn't getting any excessive spending money from them. The plan that summer was to earn and save as much as possible, so I could focus on my college studies without being too stressed or needing any larger side gigs during the school year. It was better to take an extra job now. So, while we oiled houses during the day, Griff and I also spent our late afternoons working with another contractor just down the street from us in Squaw Valley. That guy was determined to get a full day's labor out of us each afternoon. The days on the jobsite were long and the work was challenging, but Griff and I didn't care about that. The money we were pulling in gave us an exhilarating sense of freedom.

When it came time for college, I had a thorny problem: my grades. The building bug had bitten me hard. I didn't want to be that guy staining houses and toting five-gallon buckets of rocks until I retired. The architecture school at UC Berkeley was the dream answer. Not only was Berkeley's architecture program among the top ten in the world, but the campus was close to home.

Since I hadn't burned up the honor roll in high school, the easiest path forward was following my friends to CU Boulder. I was admitted into a program called Environmental Design, which meant I'd have to figure out my formal architectural education later. Colorado had mountains and adventure, making it an easy choice, even though it was a nineteen-hour drive from home.

9

An Italian Adventure

Things turn out best for people who make the best of the way things turn out.

—John Wooden

By the time classes started in the fall of 1982, Boulder, Colorado had become a celebrity city. Since 1978, it had been the setting for the ABC sitcom *Mork & Mindy*, starring Robin Williams and Pam Dawber. The quirky show was about an eccentric alien named Mork who formed an unlikely friendship with the down-to-earth Mindy. The show was a big hit, increasing tourism and out-of-state enrollment at the university. There were so many California students at CU Boulder that we affectionately called the institution the "University of California at Boulder." I even capitalized on the catchy phrase by screen-printing it in collegiate lettering onto high-quality T-shirts, selling them to local stores.

A campus full of laid-back, sun-soaked West Coasters, tourists, and TV crews was the perfect petri dish for a party school. I even pledged and later joined the Chi Psi fraternity. Several unique experiences ensued, few of which I'm proud. I could list several of them, but it would be easier for readers to just google "typical frat life" then select "images"—you get the picture. The experience was certainly entertaining, though it undeniably took focus away from the academics my parents were investing in. As time went on, I realized it probably wasn't my scene, and I began to feel restless.

During the summer of 1983, I was able to work for the architecture firm Robinson Mills & Williams back in San Francisco. I'd known David Robinson's daughter in high school, and after she introduced us, he became a mentor of sorts, eventually offering me a short summer internship. Keep in mind, I was more of an office hand than an architect's assistant. Regardless, I got firsthand experience of what went on in the business. Architecture had remained my passion for several years already.

By the time I was halfway through my sophomore year, I knew I wanted something different. My grades were slipping because my heart wasn't engaged in most of my environment design classes, even though the mountains were beautiful and the social scene was buzzing. I longed for more focus and purpose—something that felt meaningful and connected to the future I envisioned. As much as I loved the outdoor adventures Boulder offered, I knew deep down that my true path was elsewhere. It was time to head back to San Francisco.

I packed up and left CU Boulder after completing fall semester my sophomore year and spent the following spring semester at City College of San Francisco. My plan was as simple as it gets: to work hard and keep my sights set on transferring to Berkeley's undergraduate architecture program. I received sage advice from an old friend of mine, Brad Onorato, that if I went to City College and completed some prerequisite classes in architecture, I would be admitted into Berkeley's program. None of this would have been possible without Brad. I was accepted for the fall of 1984 to the school I knew was the right place.

My grades and course credits were finally where they needed to be. My concentrated architecture studies were on campus in Wurster Hall. Here's an irony for you: I was taught how to design beautiful, world-class structures inside of a building of raw, unadorned concrete that loomed over the campus like something Stalin dreamed up. Wurster's style of architecture is aptly named Brutalism. Maybe that was the point: The building made every student's design, no matter how bad, feel worthy of an American Institute of Architects Gold Medal.

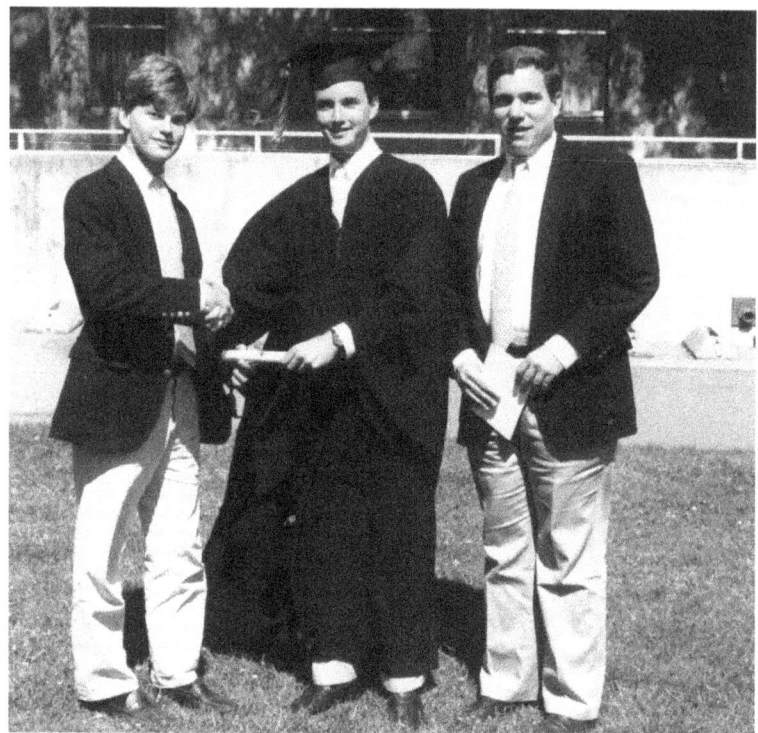

UC Berkeley, Graduation Day, 1986, with brother Chris and friend
Brad Onorato, who helped me navigate the admissions process

Despite Wurster Hall's vibe, I felt I was exactly where I needed to be. Architecture fascinated me, and I studied it in earnest. My days were a blur of sketching, model-making, and design theory. The challenge excited me. How a vision could be transformed from a rough sketch into something tangible felt instinctive to me. Since I'd been a part of that construction process during my summers in Lake Tahoe, I may have had a distinct advantage over my fellow students at Berkeley. Most of them had never picked up a hammer, let alone witnessed a foundation getting poured or a framed wall being lifted into place.

In the evenings, I had a job parking cars at Fiore de Italia, a bustling restaurant in San Francisco—and a bustling restaurant with valet parking meant decent tips. It wasn't long before I had saved enough to buy a Yamaha CA50 scooter. After class each day, I zipped around Berkeley feeling pretty cool—just like the Italians on their Vespas. The scooter was powerful enough to give me the freedom to navigate the Berkeley Hills with ease. As an added bonus, I could always find a parking space for the motor scooter on the Upper East Side, where I lived.

Fiore de Italia wasn't the only job I had in college. Like the summer of staining houses and *Cool Hand Luke*-style chain gang work, I had a knack for finding oddball ways of making money. One of my more unique opportunities came thanks to my friend Greg Applegarth. He worked as the house boy at the Pi Beta Phi sorority at Berkeley. As fate would have it, this was the same sorority my mother had pledged and joined twenty-two years earlier. Greg managed to bring a few of us on as hashers, which meant we served meals to the sorority girls and cleaned up the kitchen afterward. In return, we were fed well and even got a few coveted invitations to sorority dances and parties. It was an unexpected perk, adding another layer to the mix of experiences that shaped my Berkeley years. For the first time, I balanced my social life, school, and work with what felt like effortless ease. Confident and energized, I knew I was finally hitting my stride.

That same sense of adventure and openness to new experiences continued to guide me. Right before graduation, I found myself on the verge of another unexpected opportunity, this time far beyond campus. I had just finished a senior graduate course in architecture taught by a visiting professor, Roberto Pirzio-Biroli. He was from the Veneto region of northern Italy, and his passion for architectural history and restoration was infectious. Roberto casually mentioned at the end of the semester that if anyone wanted to work with him that summer, they should let him know. To my surprise, and his, I was the only one who took him up on the offer. I thought half of the class would jump at the chance to go to Italy, but it seemed I was the one destined for the adventure. After all, as part of my liberal arts core curriculum, I had already taken several semesters of Italian.

So, I booked a flight to Europe, ready for the experience of a lifetime. How could I not be inspired by the promise of architectural discovery in a land where it had flourished for centuries? I had visions of ancient buildings and groundbreaking projects swirling in my mind—surely, I would be inspired to design award-winning buildings with that background. But Italy, like any great adventure, had its own plans for me.

John Baker

When I arrived, things didn't go as planned. For two weeks, Roberto was nowhere to be found. I repeatedly called him at the number he provided. I even wrote a letter to the address I had for him. There was no reply. I wondered if he'd come to an untimely end or walked into the Italian version of the Bermuda Triangle. It was a strange, unnerving introduction to a country whose language I knew only so well and dwindling funds to keep me waiting. At the end of the second week, I wondered if I'd made a mistake.

I could've booked a flight home just as easily as I'd gotten one there, but I put those thoughts out of my mind. What would be the point of traveling halfway around the world if I gave up now? After making phone contact with Roberto, he instructed me to go study the works of Andrea Palladio, one of the most famous Italian classical architects in the world. Over the next couple of weeks, this led me to seek out the libraries in Venice to help with my studies and to tour around the city to see his works. I even took a day-long excursion to Padua, Palladio's birthplace. All of this was to prepare me for what I hoped would be a project with Roberto.

Frustrated that Roberto had still not come into Venice to meet with me, I became determined to find him. I finally tracked him down at his family's villa about an hour outside Venice. I showed up unannounced. To Roberto's credit, he greeted me warmly—though I could tell he hadn't expected me to take coming to Italy so seriously. Eventually, Roberto and I made our way to Venice. Surprisingly, he was well connected to the president of the province of Venice, setting me up with a project that was far more rewarding than I ever imagined.

I was assigned to the Isola San Servolo, a small island in the Venetian lagoon. Originally, the island held a monastery in the eighth century. A thousand years later, a military hospital stood on the bones of the monastery. The Italian army abandoned the hospital in the nineteenth century, and the facility was used as an insane asylum, or *manicomio*, for over a century. The asylum closed in the 1970s, leaving the island mostly abandoned and eerie, with only a few remaining inhabitants and crumbling buildings as reminders of its somber past. My task was to document the architecture of this decaying place. The buildings stood as mere shadows of their former selves. The empty halls and forgotten rooms were filled with the stories of people who had been isolated from the world.

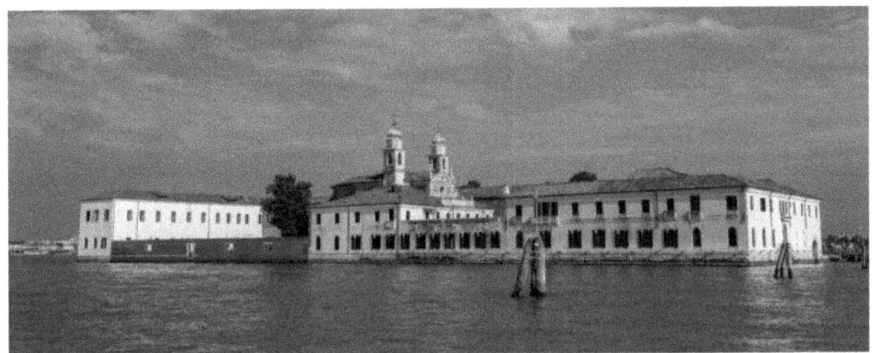

San Servolo, Venice, Italy

For months, while living in nearby Venice in student housing, I worked on the island with a small team, documenting the site and sharing meals with a few of the remaining residents who still tended the gardens. We measured room dimensions, recorded architectural details, and created archives that we hoped would one day guide a full restoration. The work was slow and methodical but quietly satisfying. There, in the shadow of Venice, I began to understand the patience it takes to truly read a building—and the care required to bring it back to life.

Roberto's vision for San Servolo wasn't just a dream or a pity project. Today, the island has been transformed into a vibrant hub. The same buildings now house the Venice International University, a museum, and the prestigious International College of Ca' Foscari University. Every time I think back to those long days on the island, I feel a sense of pride, knowing that I had a small hand in preserving a piece of history that now stands proud once again.

After my summer in Venice, I returned to the States and decided to try out the "real" working world—complete with a desk job and a boss. During that time, my friend Beau and I reconnected and moved into a makeshift "one-bedroom" apartment in Sausalito with a third roommate, Amy Krajewski. Our housing was more creative than conventional: I slept on the enclosed sun porch, Beau took over the old laundry room, and

Amy shared the actual bedroom with her boyfriend, Herman. Somehow, we made it all work.

From 1986 to 1987, over an eighteen-month stretch, I worked my first official job for a man named Fred Karen. He ran an architecture and real estate development office based in Oakland, with properties scattered across the Bay Area. I came into the job expecting to work closely with the architects, hoping they'd show me the ropes so I could contribute to minor design changes or additions. Instead, I found myself serving as Fred's property manager. My workspace was a small, windowless office just off the lobby—strategically placed, so that his assistant could keep tabs on me. Still, it didn't take long for me to recognize that working for Fred was an opportunity in disguise.

Fred was a visionary. In the late 1980s, he pioneered the conversion of old multi-story warehouses like the Serta Mattress manufacturing warehouse into live-work lofts, a novel concept in commercial real estate at the time. I soon understood I was on the cutting edge of redevelopment. I had the benefit of making weekly site visits to his properties. He owned several prominent properties, including 175 Bluxome Street in San Francisco, the original headquarters of Banana Republic. This old brick building featured large arched windows and high ceilings, giving it a distinctive look. The coolest part, however, was the old wooden freight elevator, complete with a creaky, slatted wooden gate—the kind no longer permitted in commercial buildings today. Another building I managed for Fred was a multi-floor warehouse at 100 Harrison Street in San Francisco. Winterland Productions was the anchor tenant. It didn't get any cooler than managing a property for the company that made all the merchandise for the Grateful Dead.

My duties quickly made me Fred's right-hand man. I became his day-to-day representative, handling lease negotiations and managing tenant improvements. Through this work, I found that dyslexia gave me a superpower. I could read and understand contracts with a clarity I didn't think was possible. For some reason, I started reading some contracts backward. Not like a mirror image but starting from the signature line and working my way up. It made more sense to me that way, and I found many errors and incongruities that even Fred's legal team had missed.

Heart of the Journey

The more responsibility Fred put on my shoulders, the more empowering my role became. I stepped into meetings and knew I had the authority to make decisions. I was making a difference, and that made me want to stay. It was a heady experience for someone a year out of college, and the work came naturally to me. With little effort, I gained respect in the business. That fueled my confidence that real estate might one day be where I'd return. It's not often that someone is lucky enough to fall into a business or trade they love, but I knew one thing for certain: I had always been intrigued by architecture and buildings.

After a year and a half of working with Fred, I felt the pull of adventure once again. There's a comfort in regularity and routine, but after all, doesn't familiarity breed contempt? I had figured out, at the early age of twenty-four, that I wanted to chart my own course in life, not just be under the watchful eye and security of an employer. I wasn't running away from the inevitability of needing full-time employment. In fact, I was running toward something far greater: the entrepreneurial mindset that I believe allowed for a work-life balance. If I didn't have the confidence of knowing I could find the monetary success I desired in my field, I might not have taken on the next adventure.

It was the fall of 1987, and some of my friends had taken a gap year between graduation and work. I saw this as my deferred gap year, a chance to hit pause on the work thing and chase a dream. *The real estate world will always be there,* I said to myself. At that moment, I was ready for something different and a bit daring.

Teaching at the Jackson Hole Ski School was on my radar. The thought of spending a winter in the mountains felt like the perfect next step. Not necessarily for a long-term career, but as another adventure I felt compelled to pursue. Working for the ski school wasn't as simple as it might sound. Although my boyish charms had secured me a position at Big Red's Chicken & Spaghetti, they didn't cut it here. I had to be more than a proficient skier and instructor. I had to be outstanding—and there were hundreds of other candidates who wanted the same thing I did.

I spent the month prior making phone calls and planning my move to Jackson Hole. In 1987, YouTube videos on "how to make the perfect stem christie" did not exist. I also didn't have much of a plan B. What if I didn't make it? Would I end up waiting tables or having to return home? The thought crossed my mind more than once, but I kept pushing forward. I packed everything I owned into my small, rear-wheel-drive BMW 2002—a car I'd bought after admiring Griff's a couple of years earlier—and planned my route to the Grand Tetons.

Luck was on my side in more ways than one. My high school friend, Katie Knick, had the same idea. She and her boyfriend Derick were planning to move to Jackson, and she decided to ride with me to get a head start on finding housing. I'll never forget how we crammed her belongings into every nook and cranny of my car. We waved goodbye to her parents and off we went, two friends chasing a mountain dream, relying solely on our luck, talent, and resourcefulness.

When we arrived in Jackson Hole, reality set in. The application process, training, and on-mountain exam were no joke. It wasn't just about skiing well. The Jackson Hole Ski School was run by Josef "Pepi" Stiegler, the 1964 Olympic gold medalist of slalom skiing. He had high standards, and he personally tested us. Pepi took us up the tram one day and said in his thick Austrian accent, *"Point your skis straight down zee 'ill and see how long you can last."* Then, he led the way. Watching Pepi carve perfect, controlled turns down Rendezvous Bowl at high speeds was mesmerizing. None of us could keep up, but I was proud to be one of the standouts.

The school wasn't just looking for fast skiers, though. I think chasing Pepi down the slope was a way to test our nerves and resolve. Pepi and his team wanted instructors with solid skiing ability who also had social skills and could be good teachers. At the end of the selection process, Katie, Derick, and I were fortunate enough to be offered jobs. We signed the lease on a condo and settled in. There wasn't much to do with our limited budgets except wait for more snow to fall that winter.

When the skiers finally started arriving for the season, I had a rude awakening. Wyoming winters are no joke, and with my rear-wheel drive car sidelined for the season, we were left to hitchhike to work each day. One frigid morning, a man in a pickup truck pulled over and waved us in—but when we opened the passenger-side door, he motioned toward the truck bed instead. It was about −5°F that morning—and with the wind chill, it had to be closer to −20°F. You could have been dressed like an arctic explorer, and the cold still would have seeped into your bones. None of us complained. Katie never said, "Why the hell did we decide to do this?" We all wanted to be there. The cold couldn't dampen the excitement of living and working in such a legendary place.

At some point that season, after peeking over the edge on many occasions, I made my decision: I was going to jump into Corbet's Couloir. Infamous as America's scariest ski slope, the narrow slot entrance was flanked by sheer rock faces and crowded with onlookers who were sizing each other up. Every second of the run promised a heart-pounding rush far greater than the adrenaline I'd felt biking alongside my dad with logging trucks roaring past at high speeds.

Some saw skiing Corbet's as a rite of passage. Others called it reckless, unnecessary. I wasn't trying to prove anything to Pepi or anyone else. It was just a thrill I couldn't resist, a challenge I believed was just within my wheelhouse.

I slid my Kastle 195 ski tips just over the icy cornice edge, then slid back, giving myself time to reconsider. Moving them a bit to the left offered me a better entry area. After sitting with the sick, sinking feeling in my gut, I finally hung my ski tips over the edge with forced confidence, processing all the possible outcomes as I waited for my turn to drop in. The fear of accidentally going off the edge was still a factor, and voices inside my head were trying to reason with the outside hoots and hollers of the other thrill seekers playing the same game I was. Everyone had their own coping mechanisms, and I needed to use mine.

There was no particular order to dropping into Corbet's, but it appeared I was up next.

"One, two, three . . ."

I launched into the air.

There's no rehearsal for free-falling at 40 mph, landing on a 50-degree slope, and instantly battling for control in an area confined by rock walls. The world blurred. My instincts kicked into high alert. Each turn was a fight to stay upright.

But somehow, I pulled it off.

And I lived to tell the story.

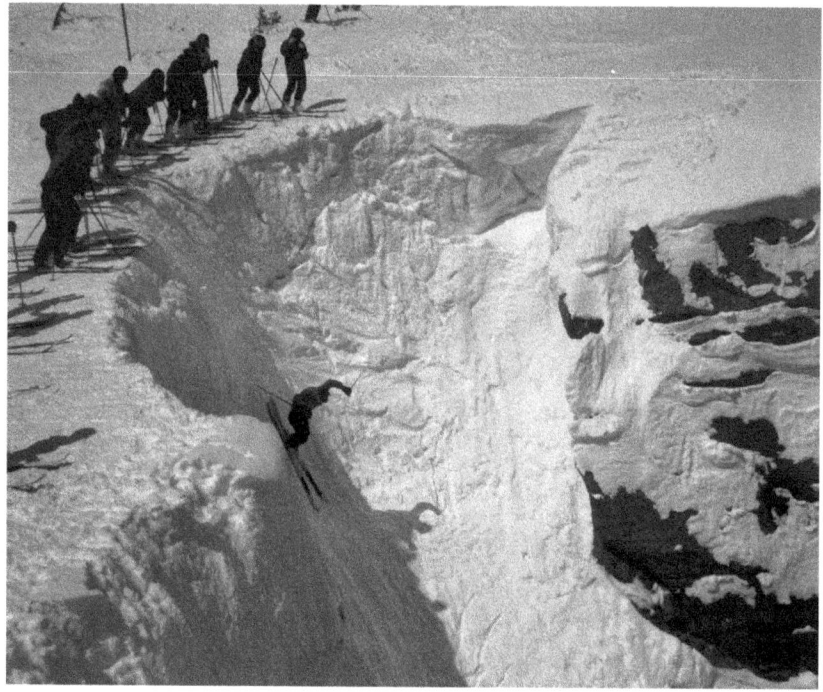

That's me, launching into Corbet's Couloir

However, I felt my most impressive accomplishment that winter wasn't conquering the famous Corbet's Couloir several times but logging 163 days of skiing that year on Jackson Hole's mountain. Each frigid day was full of adventure, challenge, and rewarding teaching experiences. More than anything, it was a season of living fully in the moment, embracing the unknown, and proving to myself that I could take on whatever came next.

10

New Zealand Awaits

Spoiler alert . . . everything will be okay.
—Bill Murray

I had fully expected to rejoin the "working world" doing something within my wheelhouse after the winter at Jackson Hole. I was young, but not delusional enough to think I could make a living and be satisfied as a ski instructor—there were only so many days you could be Peter Pan. I personally felt I needed to become a more productive member of society.

But I'd wait to grow up another day.

My spirit of adventure wasn't ready to let up; I had at least one more in me and just enough savings before I had to worry about filling out requests for time off. In the spring of 1989, I embarked on an unforgettable journey biking through New Zealand with Griff Towle. Griff had come a long way from staining houses with me at Lake Tahoe. He'd wrapped up law school and had three weeks of freedom before his job started at a prestigious law firm in San Francisco.

Griff wasn't only a savvy entrepreneur; he also had a brilliant legal mind. When I heard the news, I knew Griff would want an adventure to celebrate his new job. It had to be something epic to close out this chapter before he settled into the grind of a legal career. I don't exactly remember how we decided on New Zealand, but once we had the idea, there was no going back. As fate would have it, Griff went on to spend his entire career at that firm. I know this because we remain close friends to this day.

A tourist book on New Zealand would guide our initial travel planning. From the book, we gathered that rain would play a big part in the experience, so having proper rain gear was essential. Additionally, all our clothing would need to be placed in plastic bags to keep it dry before we placed it in our bike's side panniers. We packed everything up, cramming extra gear into the used bicycle boxes before wrapping them with extra duct tape and some hope. The ticketing staff at the airport casually slid the bike boxes into the oversized baggage area, giving us little confidence that our bikes would actually arrive.

In 1989, flying with something like a mountain bike wasn't much easier than it is today, but all the stress of preparation melted away as we got onboard our flight to Auckland. Griff and I were as equipped as two eager twenty-somethings could be. By that, I mean we were fully prepared to ride into whatever lay ahead. When we landed in Auckland, we lugged our gear to a quiet spot near the terminal exit, tore open the boxes, and began piecing the bikes back together, eventually pedaling our way downtown.

Auckland's skyline reached upward, a mix of modern architecture against a deep-blue harbor dotted with sailboats. For those unfamiliar with New Zealand's geography, the country has an incredibly diverse landscape made up of two main islands, North and South. Though part of the same country, North and South Island each have a character of their own. We had a loose plan to circumnavigate part of the North Island, working our way inland to where the indigenous Māori lived, then down the west coast of the South Island. Keep in mind that this was 1989 and New Zealand has a low population density. So, once we pedaled out of Auckland, we were on our own until we found a remote town or village. There were no cell phones, and our equivalent of GPS was a paper map and compass, so we needed to remain flexible.

The North Island was our introduction, where the heartbeat of New Zealand's modern world meets the echoes of its ancient heritage. From the moment we ventured out, it was clear we were in a place where urban life and wilderness coexisted in an easy rhythm. However, after our first week on the road with our mountain bikes, we were anxious for the real wilderness that awaited on the South Island. We booked a short flight from Wellington on the North Island to Nelson, a town nestled at the northern tip of the South Island. The South Island has more rugged and untouched landscapes than its northern counterpart; it is where much of the *Lord of the Rings* movies were later filmed. As soon as we touched down in Nelson, we were ready to explore its pristine wilderness.

From Nelson, we pedaled into the damp but breathtakingly beautiful Abel Tasman region and onto the Heaphy Track. This was true, untamed wilderness, the likes of which I had never seen before. The only comparison to the experience I could think of was what it might have felt like to be one of the first to stumble upon the Hawaiian Islands before they were touched by development. Tropical wilderness stretched as far as the eye could see, all along narrow single-track trails meant more for hiking than for cycling. Griff and I quickly learned that our bikes weren't exactly suited for these conditions.

One of the most challenging things to navigate was New Zealand's suspension bridges. Many of these bridges spanned across rushing rivers and were barely wide enough for one person, so we had no option but to hoist our bikes and gear across separately. We often had to wade through rivers, struggling to keep our belongings dry—staying dry ourselves was a lost cause. Yet, in those muddy, challenging moments, we found joy in the struggle. There was a raw exhilaration in pushing through such rugged, untouched terrain.

We worked our way down the rainy west coast of the South Island, a journey marked by vistas I still struggle to describe fully. Once beyond the wilderness, there were the small, sleepy towns of Westport and Greymouth, where we'd gather minimal supplies and chat with locals. The untouched Fox Glacier took our breath away, along with the rugged coastline that seemed to carry the soul of the land itself. Our meals were as simple as our lodgings—usually some local whitefish and canned vegetables, shared as we dried our clothing and rested our weary legs from hours of pedaling.

Somewhere in all that effort of carrying our bikes through freezing rivers, grinding up slippery hills, and peeling off wet socks at the end of every long day, I began to understand something that would last: comfort rarely teaches you anything. It's the struggle, the laughing through soaked clothes and sore legs, and the bonding that burns itself into memory. That's the part of a journey that ends up meaning the most.

The end of our journey brought us to the gorgeous fjords of Milford Sound and the lively town of Wanaka. Here, we decided to trade in our bikes for skis, and I was eager to feel some snow under my feet again. We scraped together enough money to rent some gear and booked an affordable helicopter ride into the Harris Mountains. It was the tail end of New Zealand's winter season, so there were year-end bargains to be had. We spent the day carving through the fresh powder of untouched snowfields beneath a blue sky. When I say blue, I don't mean the blue you get in the States—it could be the cleaner air or the sun hitting the atmosphere at a different angle, but the sky's hue seems more brilliant there.

By the end of those three weeks, New Zealand had given us everything we could have wanted from an adventure and more. Griff and I would soon fly back to the States, where he'd begin his long legal career, and I'd carry forward the memories of wading through rivers with a bike over my head, living off canned food, and finding freedom in the wild expanse of New Zealand's South Island. It was an adventure that marked, for both of us, what we thought of as a farewell to our carefree youth before life's responsibilities set in.

***

One of the key secrets to a fulfilling life that many people either overlook or fail to embrace is the realization that there's no specific moment when you truly cross into an adult frame of mind. There's no rule that says there's no more adventure when you start a career and take on the task of supporting yourself and family, that crossing that threshold means no more adventure. I have my father to thank for that mindset. He balanced work and adventures quite nicely; I decided to do the same.

Mountain biking became my tether to thrill and exploration, weaving itself through my life from 1990 to 2000—and with Peggy, the final few years. Those years were a mosaic of nubby tires biting into rocky terrain while racing through the wild beauty of the western United States.

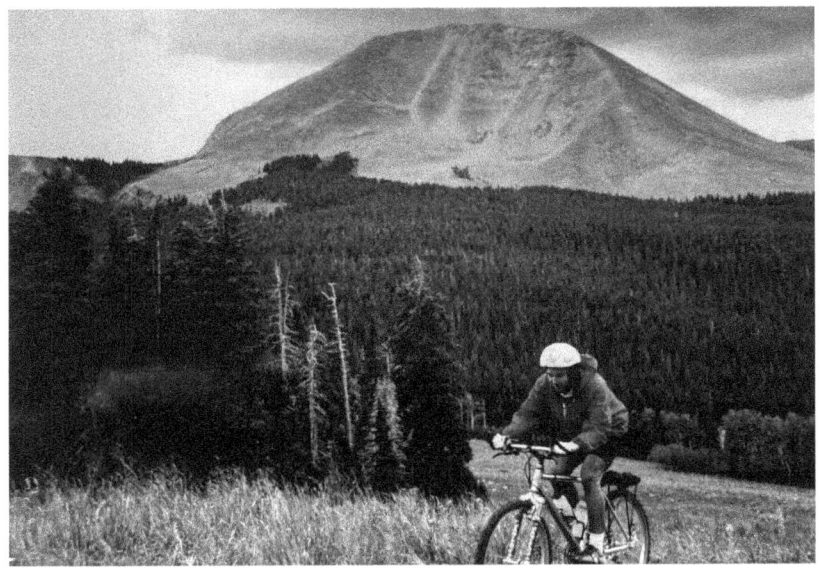

Crested Butte to Aspen, Colorado, over Pearl Pass

The mountains and trails in this region held an unspoken promise of the transcendence I'd experienced on trails in New Zealand. I chased that rush from the stark red arches of Moab's Slick Rock and Poison Spider to the steep slopes of Park City, from Crested Butte's wildflowered high meadows to Lake Tahoe's sweeping lake vistas on the Flume Trail and Mr. Toad's Wild Ride, to name a few.

When you have a career, you chase adventure when you can—that means evenings, weekends, and holidays, not waiting for the perfect bluebird conditions. If I had always waited for pretty, 72° F days with a light breeze, I wouldn't have ever gone biking. The conditions could range from blazing sun to pouring rain. Other times, it was in the chilled air of night rides—cruising through places like Marin's famed Mount Tamalpais—that I found my only time to adventure out and exercise. I'd strap on a headlamp and feel the silent rush as it unfolded under the stars, on thrill-seeking trails with names such as Tenderfoot, Repack, and Hoo-Koo-E-Koo.

11

Early Years as a GC

You work 80 hours a week so you don't have to work 40.
—Mark Cuban

My life wasn't just about cresting peaks and carving lines in the dirt during those years. My professional world was evolving, too. My foundation in architecture was beginning to morph into something more hands-on. I found my niche in general contracting (GC), which eventually sparked a vision for something bigger for later in my career: commercial real estate investment. I wanted to build spaces that felt like a natural extension of the landscape, where people could feel the same thrill I did on those mountain trails, but within four walls.

I felt that starting small was the best and maybe only way to go in my situation. There was less financial risk to dipping your toe in the water with smaller projects. The minimized risk gives you a learning laboratory to make mistakes and build your confidence for what comes next. It's easy to say that in hindsight, looking at my journey through the lens of history—but the truth is, I had no blueprint for success. I simply made thoughtful decisions and responded well to the opportunities that came my way.

After returning from my travel adventures, I worked for a small construction company in Sausalito, California. I don't recall who pointed me in this direction, but I loved architecture, buildings, and working with my hands, so why wouldn't I start at the bottom and learn how structures were actually built? Within a year, I had been asked by family and friends if I would take on side projects. Gutting and rebuilding my parents' kitchen was by far the largest and most challenging at the time. Every new venture comes with upfront costs. For me, the biggest investment was a leased Ford Ranger midsize truck, outfitted with a WeatherGuard toolbox. Inside were the Makita and Hitachi power tools I'd gradually collected—just a modest set that, until then, had been crammed into the trunk of my car.

Shortly thereafter, in 1990, I landed my first high-profile project as the prime contractor for the San Francisco Decorator Showcase Home on Vallejo Street. The showcase is a prestigious annual event in San Francisco, where top interior designers are invited to transform a luxury home—often one with historical or architectural significance—into a walk-through display of design talent. Each designer takes on a different room, and the public is invited to tour the home, with ticket sales benefiting a local charity. It's one of those rare projects that draws attention from both industry insiders and the broader community. While I've never been a fan of doing work just for the exposure, I knew the showcase had the potential to make lasting connections and kickstart my business.

Pulling up to the house on Vallejo Street in my new truck, ready and with my toolbox loaded, felt right. It was how a young and driven GC should arrive to make his mark—and the house was a blank canvas. Each room was crafted with Old World elegance. However, what changed everything for me at the showcase was meeting an interior designer named Agnes Bourne. Agnes is a force in the design world. She's celebrated for her lectures and whimsical design, and at the time, her work filled the pages of the most prestigious design publications. Luckily for me, she recognized my strong work ethic, attention to detail, and easygoing personality, traits not always common in the trades.

A group of us stood in the formal kitchen of the showcase home on Vallejo Street. If the worn and tired plaster walls could talk, they would've described the countless meals prepared by chefs and staff over the years. This was the stately kitchen I was preparing to bring back to life, with the design expertise of Agnes Bourne. Some people just have a sparkle to them, and you certainly know when they have entered the room. That was Agnes—presenting herself at the kickoff meeting in a brightly colored outfit, slightly oversized glasses, and with a sharp, whimsical eye that rarely missed a detail. She was cheerful and energetic, and she took an immediate liking to me. From the start, she trusted that I could translate her vision into reality and deliver a finished project worthy of publication. I must have done something right, because in the years that followed, she brought me in to work on her personal residence as well.

Agnes didn't just trust me with her projects. She connected me with her network. Her belief gave a credibility I couldn't have conjured alone. In fact, she told me to change the name of my business from Boardman Building to Baker Construction; Boardman was my middle name, passed down from my father's side.

"Baker is your last name, and construction is what you do—is there any other business name that makes more sense?" she asked me during one of our meetings. "You're the boss, and your name should be on the side of your truck." Her comments set me on a path that seemed to stretch out infinitely ahead.

With every new project I snagged in the Bay Area, I was building not just spaces but a name for myself. Both metaphorically and literally, I had a seat at the adult table—though I hadn't entirely planned it. Throughout 1991, I took on an assortment of projects, most of which stemmed from the showcase house (and my relationship with Agnes, more specifically). She had me work on her beautiful home, which was also on Vallejo Street in San Francisco, just down the street from the showcase.

No sooner was Agnes' renovation complete than she sold the home to Jane and Joel Rosenberg, cheerfully telling them, "John is the contractor that comes with the house!" Like Agnes, the Rosenbergs had whimsical taste in design and offered up a steady stream of interesting projects. These ranged from creating a wood-paneled cozy nook off their top floor media room to replacing windows and structurally bracing the garage. The work was varied and hands-on—exactly the kind of experience a young contractor needed to grow. But it wasn't just the detailed work that helped shape my career. It was the relationships—the trust, the collaboration, the chance to deliver something personal and lasting. The Rosenbergs remain the most

Heart of the Journey

unique and fun-loving couple I've ever had the pleasure of working with. Their generosity and trust extended beyond our projects together and even led to me house-sitting for them on several occasions.

My contracting work continued into 1992, with more excitement and on-the-job training. I had also assembled a good crew of guys, one of whom was named Mike Coakley. Mike and I decided to buy a fixer-upper in Park City, Utah, of all places. At the time, I could hardly believe we had the nerve to think we could pull it off, but something had shifted in me. With each job, I was gaining both experience and confidence—the kind that pushes you to take big leaps. In short order, we were able to get the financing, close on the purchase, remodel, and find short-term renters throughout our first winter. My mother even came out to Park City once construction was complete to help add those special "motherly" touches like bedding, kitchen essentials, and overall décor.

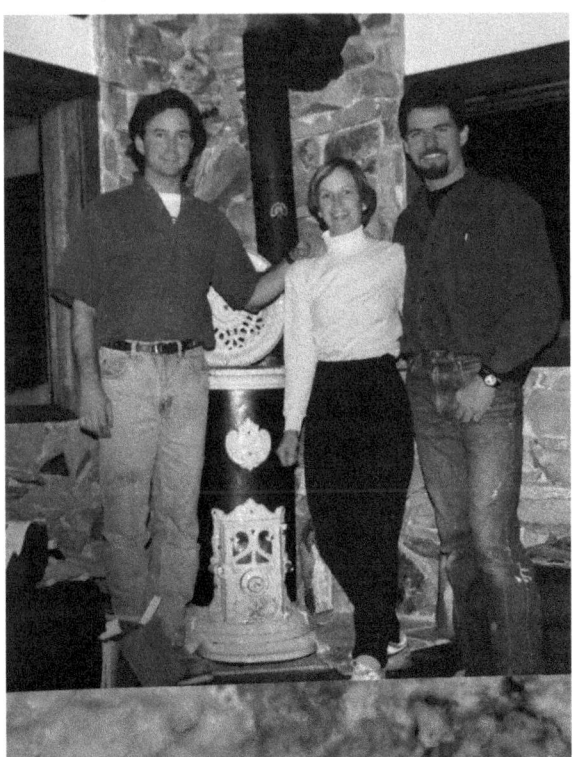

**Our own Park City fixer-upper,
with Mom and Mike Coakley, 1992**

My first project in San Francisco later that year was Café Centro, which I was to help take from raw shell to a vibrant coffee house and café. It was in the heart of South Park, a charming location south of Market Street. The client was Greg Applegarth, whom I'd known since Stuart Hall Grammar School and had previously worked with at the Pi Phi sorority house at Berkeley. Café Centro demonstrated, yet again, that what I was doing was more than a construction job. It was my first opportunity to help shape a space in a city I loved, using my hands, vision, and relationships to bring something new to life. Remarkably, this café is still thriving more than thirty years later, a testament that some places, and the memories we make in them, are worth sharing and returning to.

As time went on and I stepped back to take in the finished projects, my conviction grew. My opportunity for bigger and better things happened that same year, in late 1992, when a mutual friend introduced me to Gavin Newsom and Billy Getty. The future governor of California and J. Paul Getty's grandson were chasing a dream of their own. The duo carved out their corner of the hospitality world with PlumpJack, a name destined to become iconic in San Francisco's restaurant and hotel scene. Their ambition, like mine, was steeped in the idea of experiences. All three of us wanted to build places where people would make memories that would be talked about for years to come. Newsom and Getty were looking for someone to help bring their vision to life, starting with their flagship PlumpJack locations on Fillmore Street.

1992 was a busy year, as I was also asked by a good friend and workmate, Launce Gamble, to take on a major gut and renovation of a home he'd purchased on Potrero Hill. Not only did we take the entire house down to the studs, but we also excavated under the house to add a large garage—and there were times the house was teetering above the ground. The building inspector showed up one Friday afternoon for a framing inspection and candidly reported, "With the expected weekend winds, we might find the home collapsed by Monday morning. It would be wise of you to add some sheer bracing in short order." It was one of those lucky times where I felt like I'd dodged a bullet. The lesson was learned and noted for future projects.

At the time, I was not only the general contractor for Launce's renovation—I was also wearing the "hardhat" of a carpenter. One day, while reframing the roof, I made my second—and expensive—wrong cut sawing some roof joists. In another transformative moment, Launce offered some keen advice. He looked over and, in his tactful way, said, "You should really be out doing what you're good at: overseeing our other projects and securing our next jobs." I took it a bit personally, but he was spot-on. What I didn't realize at the time is that it was a *defining moment*. In fact, I was better at the salesmanship role and at overseeing the projects with a critical, high-level vision.

Launce later went on to be an invaluable assistant on the PlumpJack Inn project in Squaw Valley, and, of course, remains a good friend to this day. Listening is an invaluable skill, and when he speaks, he's someone whose words I still pay attention to.

I undertook what would become the most fascinating project of my young career in late 1992, going into 1993. I was hired to construct a freestanding observatory for Timothy Ferris, the renowned and outspoken Berkeley professor of astronomy. The Rocky Hill Observatory was designed to have Mr. Ferris's office on the ground floor, plus a second level with a sliding roof that would open to expose the telescope to the night sky and stars beyond. I was pleased and surprised to be selected as his contractor, though I had received an excellent referral. Your best referrals are word-of-mouth, so if you can please people, there's no end in sight.

Building the Rocky Hill Observatory was no small feat—it was my first ground-up project on a hillside, in a remote corner of Sonoma County. From the start, I was all in. My dedication ran deep, even by my own standards; I pitched a tent under a lone oak tree on the property and camped there for the duration of the project, determined to stay close to ensure that every detail was done right. That kind of hands-on commitment became a hallmark of my early career. To this day, I'm still amazed at how we pulled off coordinating subcontractors and material deliveries without the help of cell phones.

This project coincided with the time I started dating Peggy. I'm not sure her father would have approved, if he'd been keeping close tabs on her, but she came up one Friday evening for a nice dinner in the nearby town of Glen Ellen and a sleepover in my tent. If that wasn't confidence and trust in me, I'm not sure what is.

After completing the observatory and Launce's home, and while working on the PlumpJack restaurant project, I became disillusioned with the city and its politics. I needed to set my sights elsewhere and take my show on the road, to go some place that welcomed thoughtful development and progress instead of resisting it. A simpler place, with fresh air and green open spaces—places like Glen Ellen and Lake Tahoe, which I'd visited frequently but never dreamed of living in. It seemed ski towns were where the action was in the '90s—there was skiing in winter and mountain biking in summer, and they were otherwise generally "open for business," full of young, likeminded, and healthy people.

In my professional life, it felt like I had a dual personality. I had one foot in commercial construction and another in residential development—though had I not straddled that fence, I might never have met Peggy, the person who later became my greatest support and lifeline.

12

Code Blue

Courage is fear holding on one more minute.
—George S. Patton Jr.

Friday, April 26, 2024, 2:55 a.m.

In the pediatric wing of the ER, my eyes were rolling back in my head and my skin was as white as a sheet of paper when the nurse called the code at 2:55 a.m. Peggy was shaking me to see if she could rouse me without doing CPR, but I was having none of it. As she would later tell me, I remained unconscious as the nurse cleared my airway and started CPR.

"John! John, honey, wake up!" The nurse started chest compressions. There was nothing else that Peggy could do, so she ran into the hall screaming as additional help came running. As the medical staff began to work on me, there was a rush to get fluids into my system, and one of the nurses squeezed another IV bag. Watching from the hallway, my wife had to briefly look away from my lifeless body. She'd watched her father get CPR and couldn't bring herself to associate that same memory with me.

A nurse came up to her trying to make small talk, first asking how we knew each other and where we were from. Peggy doesn't do small talk when conditions are normal, so I can only imagine how that went. While she still couldn't look at me, the nurse informed my wife in broad strokes what was happening—namely, that they'd been able to find a pulse. "They aren't using the crash cart, so that's a good sign," she told Peggy.

How could this happen to him? He's only sixty, Peggy thought, trying to make sense of the senseless event playing out before her. The nurse didn't have any answers but did her best to comfort my wife, but even that was short-lived as the code team finally funneled out of the room. Only the nurse who called the code and a man who was presumably a doctor remained by my side. Then, something in her snapped.

"What the hell did you give him?" my wife spat at the nurse. "You almost killed my husband! You're going to have to work really hard for me not to move him to Stanford Hospital."

I don't blame her for going off. Had I known what was happening, I probably would've had some choice words, too. The doctor shot the nurse a look that said, *What the hell is she going on about?* It was the silent shorthand of someone who had no interest in talking Peggy off a ledge; he glanced at her but said nothing.

"His heart didn't stop," the nurse said flatly. "I called the code because I couldn't find a pulse. It keeps going up and down, but we'll figure out what's wrong with him."

The medical staff continued to come in and out of the room every ten minutes or so, checking on me. Peggy stayed by my side, watching me and trying to be cautiously optimistic about my situation. Once I was a tad more coherent and able to make eye contact with her, she leaned in close, brushing my hair back into place with her hand.

"Don't leave me—you can't leave me!" she said, as she lightly rubbed my arm and my legs, providing touch, which is my love language. She wanted to show love to me in a way I could feel and that meant the most to me, even if I wasn't fully aware of what was going on.

Once I was finally stabilized—at least for the time being—the nurse checked my chart on the computer and shared the results from the bloodwork taken earlier in triage. She informed Peggy that I was septic and that we wouldn't be going home for a few days. That conversation triggered a memory—and an aha moment.

While the nurse was questioning how I contracted sepsis, the memory floated to the forefront of my brain about swimming in the ocean earlier in the week and getting stung by a jellyfish. So, I casually mentioned it while the nurse and Peggy were in conversation as the doctor was bedside, reviewing my chart. Why it happened at this moment, I really have no idea; my body was failing me, and the medical team was too busy keeping me stable to truly entertain the idea. Still, this new information lurked in the background as I drifted in and out of awareness—and it must have made it into the notes on my chart, because it did come up later.

What I did know, regardless of my level of awareness, was that Peggy looked surprised when I mentioned the sting, almost as if I had deliberately kept that information from her. But she quickly let go of any irritation toward me, either assuming I wasn't making sense or that I hadn't mentioned it days earlier because it didn't seem important. We'd hopefully have time to play the husband-and-wife "I told you about that," "No, you didn't!" game later.

Now, it was the doctor's turn to share necessary information. He spoke slowly and clearly, as if every word he said were a step into a minefield. "We're going to put a central line in his neck for ease of administering medication to keep his blood pressure stable. There's a blood pressure cuff on him that will periodically take a reading. We'll know at all times what his blood pressure is. The nurse is going to put an oxygen mask on his face. Now, I'm going to ask you to step out while we prep him for the central line."

Peggy left the room, thankful to at least have a short-term plan in place. Once the central line procedure was completed, I was going to be moved to the adult ER room to be monitored while next steps regarding my foot and the mystery sepsis were being decided upon.

Before Peggy came back in, the nurse placed a sticker on my chest in the location where the CPR had been administered an hour before. Had the situation not been so grim, it would have been funny if the sticker read PRESS HERE TO START, but I'm sure the verbiage was more official sounding than that.

13

The Battle Begins

Tough times don't last, tough people do.
—Kevin Lynch

Friday, April 26, 2024, 4:30 a.m.

As fate would have it, Dr. Peter Callander, the go-to orthopedic doctor in San Francisco, had been on call at 4:30 a.m. that Friday morning when an emergency call came over the radio. All he was told was that the patient appeared to have necrotic tissue around an ankle wound, the source of which had yet to be determined. Peter loved a good mystery, so he agreed to see the patient. Before hanging up, he asked the patient's name.

"John Baker," his contact from CPMC said. It was a common enough name that Peter almost dismissed it as a coincidence. Instead, he asked, "How old is he?"

"Sixty."

"Where's he from?"

After a few clickity-clacks from a keyboard, Peter's colleague said, "Looks like Idaho, but he just flew in from Hawaii."

"Oh my God, I know this guy!" Peter exclaimed.

"What do you mean you know this guy?"

"I know this guy, we're good friends—we've known each other since we were teenagers."

Peter and I met when I was in high school; we had moved in the same social circles, so it had only been a matter of time before our paths crossed. We had quickly become friends and had stayed in touch for more than forty years, but that friendship had never been more crucially important than it was that very day. Peggy had too much on her mind to connect the dots that one of my oldest friends was an orthopedic surgeon in San Francisco when I needed emergency medical attention. Whether fate or divine intervention, my case ended up in his lap. I'm probably here today because of his watchful eye.

Typically, orthopedics handle anything having to do with bones and joints, and since my right foot was visibly swollen with purple-black dying tissue, Peter thought that a plastic surgery team should be involved in my case. Since the cause of my sepsis was still unknown, the medical team decided to do an exploratory surgery to see if they could find the cause of the infection in my skin tissue—and since it was *my foot*, Peter decided to use his connections to make sure I was getting the best care possible.

5:00 a.m.

Over the next half hour, doctors and nurses randomly showed up and asked Peggy questions. Each time, she'd ask them to remove their masks so she could more accurately hear what they were saying and read lips if necessary. Thankfully, the staff obliged once they understood Peggy's need and saw her hearing aids. During that time, she said I was semi-lucid and speaking; now, however, I can't recall any of it. Peggy wondered if any of the doctors ever talked to each other, because she'd had to retell the story of the last forty-eight hours half a dozen times.

The doctors looked at my foot and another similar wound on the back of my upper left thigh. They poked at the wound sites with gloved fingers or with ever-present, foot-long Q-tips. At this time, Dr. Gabe Kind, the top plastic surgeon in town who had been assigned to my case, placed an outline around my blistering ankle, mapping the area in an effort to keep track of the spreading. The consensus was that whatever the puncture wounds were, they had become infected, and I was in the throes of sepsis.

The phrase "becoming septic" is fairly common, but it wasn't until that day that Peggy truly comprehended its meaning. Sepsis is a dangerous condition that arises when the body's response to an infection becomes unmanageable, resulting in widespread inflammation. If left untreated, as was apparently happening to me, sepsis can cause severe damage to tissues and organs and can even lead to death. Essentially, the body turns against itself while trying to fight off the infection, which overwhelms critical systems. Immediate medical intervention is crucial, because sepsis progresses rapidly and can become fatal *within a matter of hours*. If that was happening to me, the doctors could only attribute my still being alive to my overall level of physical fitness, before the sting occurred.

Things were serious. Peggy took the few minutes of quiet we had between doctor visits to hold my hand and whisper in my ear again, "Don't leave me. You can't leave me now."

My wife was begging me not to die, and all I could do was nod.

At this moment, Peggy was likely thinking, *How am I going to tell his parents? They don't even know we're here. How am I going to tell the kids?* She had always believed I was the strong one, the one who seemed invincible to any of life's challenges, the one to hold things together, no matter what. I was the person who rarely, if ever, got hurt or sick. She saw me as someone who could handle anything that came my way, who always maintained a sense of composure and resilience. It was as if I had built an invisible shield around myself that kept me safe from the hardships others might face. So, at that moment in time, none of the situation was making sense.

***

Before coming to the hospital to check on me, Peter contacted Dr. Kind to provide him an update on my condition and to ask if Dr. Kind could work on my case. What Peter didn't realize was that Dr. Kind had already been assigned to my case—and *he* was the one to inform Peter about my septic condition. Dr. Kind's plan was to go to the apparent source of the infection, which was likely dead tissue inside my foot. My foot had now swollen to almost twice its normal size, so the source of the infection didn't take a medical degree to determine—but it would take medical instruments and multiple tests to dig into the matter.

Dr. Kind poked at the blister on my foot and ran a test to see if he could find an answer or at least a clue about what was causing my foot to swell. He really wanted to wait on surgery until he thought there was no other choice, but thanks to Dr. Savage pumping me with antibiotics several hours before, he couldn't ascertain whether it was a bacterial infection. Smart money said it was, but he'd need to get under the hood and look around.

Then, Dr. Kind hit Peter with my blood pressure issue. This was the first inkling Peter had that I was in bad shape. He asked Dr. Kind to let him know what the outcome of the surgery was.

7:30 a.m.

Things were beginning to move fast now. I was slated for a CT scan, as Dr. Kind wanted to see if any of my organs were inflamed. That could cause any one of my vital organs not to function correctly or work overtime to compensate for being enlarged. After the CT scan, I was brought back to the same ER room—where Peggy was waiting alone—to be warehoused until Dr. Kind could perform exploratory surgery on my foot. The scan didn't reveal anything alarming, or at least nothing the staff chose to share with Peggy. Trying to make sense of the situation, she quietly snapped a photo of the screen monitoring my vitals and sent it to our primary physician back home, hoping someone could translate the medical jargon into plain English.

Peggy was allowed to stick around for a bit in the ER until the surgery. For the first time, the word *amputation* was mentioned as a possible outcome for my condition. She took this moment to tell Dr. Kind, "Save the foot—save him first, but also save the foot!" She then reluctantly left my side and worked her way to the surgical waiting room.

12:00 p.m.

I can't imagine how low and lonely Peggy must have felt. There is something to be said about getting out of a stressful environment to rejuvenate. The mental space can make all the difference, even if you're worried about the unknown or not being by someone's side. It allows you to gather your thoughts, recharge, and come back with a clearer head, ready to face whatever comes next.

It's easy for me to say, but I think that's what Peggy was hoping for—a chance to breathe in silence, instead of drowning in the busy chaos inside the hospital's walls.

During exploratory surgery, the doctor made two long incisions on the top and side of my right foot. It looked like someone had run a sharp knife down the back of a plump, overcooked hot dog, leaving it unstitched and open to relieve pressure. These were created to reduce the risk of something called compartment syndrome. I later learned that the immense pressure caused by swelling restricts blood flow, in turn damaging 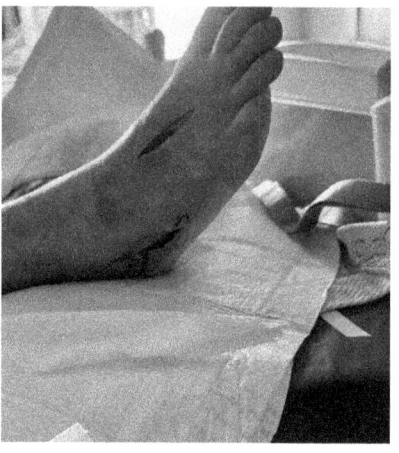 sensitive foot muscles and nerves. The incisions were necessary to prevent permanent foot damage that could compromise my ability to walk.

At this point, I was intubated due to severely compromised breathing and rapidly dropping blood pressure. I couldn't speak. The intubation tube lodged in my throat made every attempt to breathe feel mechanical, as if my body and breath no longer belonged to me. I drifted in and out, consciousness fading as the propofol took hold. I later learned that this fast-acting sedative-hypnotic was the preferred anesthesia for all my procedures, as it slowed brain activity to the point of unconsciousness. Because of my already low blood pressure, the medical team monitored my vital signs with extreme care throughout this period.

Propofol is an incredibly effective, and therefore dangerous, drug. If it sounds familiar to you or on the cusp of your memory, you've likely heard about the propofol overdose that killed Michael Jackson. Another lesser-known effect of propofol is that you don't remember anything when you're on it. Medical folks cheekily refer to it as "milk of amnesia," due to its cloudy appearance in the bottle. I can attest to the efficacy of the milk of amnesia. I already wasn't doing great with my memory from the time I got on the plane in Hawaii—but on propofol, my memory became a vast blank page on which nothing was written.

When I was finally released from this first surgery, Dr. Kind called Peggy from the waiting room to share some starkly positive news with her. Although my foot had swelled and turned grotesque colors over the last two days, there was nothing he'd seen so far that would necessitate amputation. Contrary to what we'd been originally told, Dr. Kind said he found no fistulas or necrotic tissue—yet. That was a relief. However, it still left us with more unanswered questions.

2:00 p.m.

After being my health's ringmaster, Peter anxiously awaited the report from the plastic surgeon, Dr. Kind. The report Peter received was both better than he had hoped for and more vague. Dr. Kind told Peter, "Well, it looked bad, but it didn't look horrible. There's got to be something else that's causing the sepsis besides what's happening with his foot."

2:30 p.m.

Peggy was allowed five minutes with me in recovery to give me a kiss. But after a CT scan, surgery, and more blood work, the medical staff was no closer to a diagnosis than when we got there.

After recovery, I was taken to a room in the ICU, where I laid calmly while the doctors scratched their heads over my unstable condition. I'd just gotten settled into my new room when my wife again realized, this time aloud, "God, I haven't called the kids or your parents yet. They don't know what's going on."

14

In the Deep

> *Humor is the universal solvent*
> *against the abrasive elements of life.*
> —Alan Simpson, speaking at George H. W. Bush's eulogy

Friday, April 26, 2024, 3:00 p.m.

How do you let your children know that you're in crisis and facing the unknown? What are the right words to say when you're bare-knuckle brawling with the reality of the situation? Peggy dipped her toe in those waters with a group text to our children Blair, Hayden, and Wilson:

Do you guys have a second for a call?

Wilson was the first to comment. *Yeah, sure*, he texted, followed by similar sentiments from Blair and Hayden. Peggy got everyone on a group call and launched into it: "We're in San Francisco, and your dad's in the hospital. We don't really know what's going on—he's septic, but the doctors are trying to figure it out. His blood pressure won't stay up, so they're just working on it. They're figuring it out. He has a good care team."

There's a difference between silently knowing a fact and speaking that information aloud to your children who previously had no indication that anything was wrong. Once you impart that knowledge to someone else, it becomes real. There's no turning back or hedging once you've opened your mouth. For our children, time was now defined in terms of before and after Mom called. Before, our three adult children were dealing with work issues and life's trivialities. After the call, they were facing the same unknowns as Peggy.

But uncertainty is exactly why she held off calling the kids—it wasn't that she had been ducking the call. She was just concerned about the surgery. Any surgery brings a risk, but with my blood pressure pinballing the way it was, there was a possibility it would bottom out and I wouldn't recover.

Then there was the question of my foot. For all my wife knew, as soon as the surgeon put scalpel to the skin, my foot would pop like a piñata or have to be removed. She wanted to have something solid to tell our children when I came out of surgery.

They had a million questions, and Peggy tried to answer them as best she could. The chief question was, "Should we fly to San Francisco and be at the hospital right now?"

"No, not at this point," Peggy told them. "I'll let you know what's going on. He's going to be okay."

Wilson then asked, "Do Grandma and Papa know?"

When Peggy indicated they were next on her list to call, Blair offered to take that off her plate. It took Blair a few times to reach them—they weren't chained to their phones like everyone else was, since there was little urgency in retirement. Blair finally texted my mother as a reminder to call back.

My mother freaked out the moment Blair said the word sepsis. She kept repeating, "Sepsis is really bad. It can be really bad. You can die from that!"

Blair stopped her before she could launch into an "I remember back in my day there was this boy who got sepsis . . ." story. It was as much an effort to keep her grandmother from going down a rabbit hole as it was for Blair's mental health.

"He's going to be fine," said Blair. "We're not too worried about it. I googled it, and it sounds like minor sepsis, Grandma. We're not even planning to go out there. Mom said it's fine. He'll be fine."

While Blair was talking to her grandparents, Peggy was by my side in post-op, fighting sepsis of the mind. Evolution has hardwired humans to have worst-case scenario thinking when faced with the unknown, but she refused to engage in dumpster-fire thoughts to the point that she was dousing the flames with near-toxic positivity. Being oppressively positive wasn't always Peggy's nature, but she was full-blown positive now. The doctors and nurses were telling her how sick I was, but she wasn't having any of it. Later, Peggy told me that every time someone from the medical staff had spoken to her about anything outside of blue skies and rainbows, she'd thought: *That's not an option. We're not going there. We're not thinking that. We're only doing positive thoughts now. Positive, positive, positive—no negativity, Peggy.*

5:55 p.m.

After seeing his last patients, Dr. Peter Callander arrived at CPMC. He was bedside with me in the ICU when Peggy came back into the room. This was the first time she had laid eyes on Peter and realized that he had been looking in on me remotely all day. They quickly caught up while I was zonked out. A brass band could have come into the room, and I'd have been none the wiser.

Dr. Callander checked my chart and conversed with the ICU staff assigned to me. One of the nurses wanted to wake me up. The medical team felt it was critical to wean me off the propofol to check my brain function, and so I could have a moment to see my wife and my friend Peter. Even though I wasn't in any sort of lucid state, I still recognized Peter and knew he was instrumental in my care. I looked clearly pleased to have him on my team, trying to make my hands into a heart shape like the twelve-year-old girls do on social media.

How I was able to put all of that together, and for it to be recognized by Peter, still baffles me. All I know is that I wanted my friend to know that I loved him. He got the message and set about doing everything in his power to make me well again.

7:00 p.m.

Peter or no Peter, the ICU staff kicked Peggy out at this time. Visiting hours were 10:00 a.m. to 7:00 p.m., no exceptions. It was a wise policy, as patients needed to rest and loved ones needed to recharge. Peggy didn't want to go, but she knew it was best for everyone, herself most of all. Her top priorities now were getting in touch with my brother Chris and going to bed.

Chris had been driving to Tahoe for a few days of recreation when Peggy let him know what was going on.

"Do I need to turn around and come to the hospital?" he asked.

"No, go on, I think he's going to be okay," she said. "But I'll keep you posted."

8:30 p.m.

Being mentally alert and able to make good decisions is far more important than smelling hospital sanitizer or staring at your unresponsive loved one. Maintaining a mental façade can be just as exhausting as the stress of managing a medical crisis, so don't think your love or devotion is measured in hours spent at someone's bedside. Once Peggy had contacted everyone who needed to know, she finally returned to the hotel—for the first time—to take a break from the relentless pressures. She had done everything humanly possible for me and now lay down for some well-deserved rest, though it took a while for her to fall asleep. The last time she looked at the clock before she fell asleep, it was 9:30 p.m.

15

Seven Missed Calls

—⧸⧸⟶

Pain is temporary. Quitting lasts forever.
—Kevin Lynch

Saturday, April 27, 2024, Early Morning Hours

Peggy was awoken by concussive booms reverberating against the hotel bedroom windows. She didn't know if it was an explosion or an earthquake. The only way to find out was to pull back the curtains and look outside. It took her a moment to understand that the booms and flashes in the air were fireworks from nearby Oracle Park. The Giants had pulled out a 3–0 win against the Pirates, contributing their small part to my story.

Peggy was miffed that she'd been awoken by fireworks until she looked at her phone and saw seven missed calls from the hospital, complete with voicemails. For a moment, she panicked, unable to imagine how she'd missed them. Then, she realized that years earlier, she'd set her phone to be in "do not disturb" mode after 10:00 p.m. and hadn't thought about disabling the setting in the midst of this crisis.

She began shaking so badly in fear that she almost couldn't operate the phone. I've never asked her what she was thinking, but I know even with her positive self-talk, she likely thought I was dead. She did have the presence of mind not to listen to the voicemails and called the number back immediately. Her call went to a switchboard first before starting to ring again. The answering nurse immediately launched into a flurry of questions without Peggy knowing exactly what was happening.

"We just need to ask some questions and get approvals," said the nurse in a stern voice.

"Uh, okay," Peggy replied, still trying to grasp what she was being told about my condition.

"Does he have heart issues? Is there a family history of heart disease or anything like that? Is he on heart medications?" asked the nurse.

"Well, his grandfather and great uncle had heart problems, but his heart is fine," said Peggy.

"Can we put stents in?"

Still dazed, Peggy replied, "Whatever you need to do."

"Maybe ECMO. They're taking him back now," stated the nurse.

Peggy didn't know ECMO from Elmo, but it didn't matter. Trained medical professionals were obviously going to do something to my heart. They were the experts, and I think my wife would have told them to sacrifice chicken nuggets to the deity of their choice if it would make me better.

12:15 a.m.

On the next call with a nurse, Peggy asked if she could come to the hospital and wait—she had to be close to me, even if she couldn't see me. With permission granted, she said, "I'll be right there," hanging up to call Peter for more detailed information.

I can't imagine Peter getting emergency ortho calls in the middle of the night—but what do I know? I'm a real estate guy. Whether it was seeing Peggy's number or just the shock of being jolted awake, Peter was immediately on edge as he picked up the phone. There was no preamble or polite phone etiquette. Instead, Peggy blurted out, "They're taking him back!"

Peter, as confused as Peggy was, asked, "Taking him back where?"

"They want to do a stent or something," said Peggy.

"A stent?" he asked. Knowing Peter, he was doing the mental medical calculus on what could have happened to me in a few hours that would land me in open heart surgery. He'd seen me literally five or six hours ago. My vitals were marginally fine. My blood pressure was low, but it wasn't that terrible. There was no good reason I should be having any issues with my heart.

Peggy might have thought Peter didn't understand what little information she was throwing his way and so further explained, "Well, a stent in his heart. They're talking about ECMO. Is that okay?"

After Peter's reassurance that ECMO was a good decision, Peggy headed to the hospital.

12:30 a.m.

Peggy hoped to be fully briefed on what happened to me overnight when she arrived at the hospital, but that would have to wait. Upon her arrival, she found her way through the ER and back to the large surgical waiting area. Apparently, she had to wait there alone for about two hours before she could see me.

As far as my case was concerned, the medical staff felt like they were in the middle of a *House* episode. Hugh Laurie wasn't on call Friday night, so the doctors and nurses caring for me had to put their heads together to solve the mystery of the septic guy from Hawaii.

Think about when you've got the flu or a bad cold. Your face and sinuses swell up, and the body's immune system kicks into overdrive. Extra white blood cells are created to fight the infection, and that swelling is part of the process. But here's the thing—when inflammation happens inside your body, especially near vital organs like the heart, it's a different story. The heart can get stressed. Blood flow becomes restricted. In some cases, those pressures can trigger serious complications, as in my case.

It made sense to assume the sepsis was caused by toxins released from dead tissue in my swollen foot. The problem, however, was that there was *no dead tissue.*

Heart of the Journey

3:30 a.m.

One of the brilliant heart doctors working on duty Friday night couldn't wrap her mind around my case. Everything she considered kept leading to a dead end. I'm told that when that happens in medicine, you start by ruling out the simple issues and work your way up to the more complex maladies. For some reason, this doctor wanted to start with the heart, because—as in my case—problems with the heart could present bizarre symptoms elsewhere in the body.

To rule out reasons my heart could be causing the massive swelling of my right foot and leg and creating massive dips in my blood pressure, the heart doctor ordered an electrocardiogram. Also known as EKG, the device measures the electrical activity of the heart to detect irregularities in rhythm, structure, or function. Every heart beats to pretty much the same rhythm, and an EKG essentially turns it into sheet music. If there's a sour note in the heart's music, a doctor can diagnose conditions such as arrhythmias, heart attacks, and other cardiac abnormalities.

Instead of the Boston Pops playing Beethoven, my heart was marching to the beat of electronic rave music. The EKG data showed that I was having heart failure. The most common reason a heart's rhythm gets thrown off kilter is that an artery is blocked or narrowed so much that blood flow is restricted. If that blockage is a clot, you can have chest pain, and your blood pressure goes south. If that clot breaks free and enters one of your heart valves, it's game over.

After reviewing the EKG results, the ICU doctor contacted the on-call interventional cardiologist, Dr. David Daniels. With nearly twenty years of experience, Dr. Daniels had been around the block a few times. And when he heard that someone admitted from the ER and transferred to the ICU was having a cardiac arrest, something didn't add up.

Usually, people come into the ER because they're having chest pains. They get an EKG, and either a heart issue is ruled out or they're treated for whatever heart issues they have. It's rare that someone in the ICU with an unrelated condition randomly has heart failure. In this high-stakes moment, his brain went into overdrive, mentally mapping the prioritized sequence of steps needed to save my life.

4:00 a.m.

After receiving the call, Dr. Daniels rushed to CPMC from the East Bay, making the trip in just thirty minutes—a rarity. They took me from the ICU to the catheterization laboratory, more commonly called the cath lab. There, doctors perform minimally invasive procedures to diagnose and treat heart conditions—they'll open a vein or artery in someone's neck or inner thigh to snake a scope or stent into the heart or part of the circulatory system.

Dr. Daniels shot me up with radioactive dye to see if there was any blockage causing my on-paper heart failure. There was no blockage, but my heart function was still dangerously low and deficient, which only raised more questions. Dr. Daniels was able to tell from that one scan that most of my organs were failing. My persistent low blood pressure meant that my kidneys and liver specifically weren't getting the blood flow they needed to operate.

Organs and blood are like fish and water. Organs need the oxygen and nutrients from blood to function, just like a fish filters oxygen through its gills to absorb it. You can take a fish out of the water for a short while—a handful of seconds—and it will be fine. If the fish is out of the water for too long, it will die. My liver and kidneys were on the precipice of being oxygen-starved fish.

The only rational diagnosis Dr. Daniels could make for my kidneys and liver was stress cardiomyopathy, a temporary heart condition triggered by intense physical stress. It mimics a heart attack, with symptoms like chest pain and shortness of breath, but—if dealt with quickly and properly—it is reversible, as the heart muscles recover over time.

What caused my heart condition was something to ascertain at a later time. But right now, Dr. Daniels had to do something, because I was literally dying.

16

Building More Than Dreams

*Happiness is less a destination
and more of a means of travel.*

—Anonymous

Transition is forever a part of life. We grow out of childhood and into adults. We grow personally and professionally. One day, we'll all transition into the *great beyond*. And throughout each phase of life, we have opportunities to learn about our own resilience and natural talents. In my early career, I was quickly learning that I was able to adapt to every situation that came my way, no doubt a benefit of so many outdoor adventures in my youth.

Times of business transition often lead to taking smaller pay-the-bills gigs while pursuing bigger fish. In 1991, one of those gigs landed in my lap: a modest bathroom remodel for a young lady two years younger than me named Peggy Mills—Jeanne White, an interior designer we both knew, had vouched for me, thinking I'd be a perfect fit for Peggy's modest renovation. I showed up with a tool belt, expecting a straightforward job and nothing out of the ordinary. But as often happens in construction, one thing led to another. What started with a bathroom grew into a kitchen, then some windows, then more. Each new phase meant more visits, more check-ins. Slowly, we got to know each other, and as the months wore on, fate was clearly at work behind the scenes, quietly stitching our paths closer together.

The relationships Peggy and I were in when we first met both dissolved at around the same time. There was no grand design to this—it wasn't like either of us had secretly been pining for each other and sabotaging our relationships to be together. Regardless, we started inviting each other to gatherings, one of which was a big party Peggy hosted for her twenty-seventh birthday. She had a lot of friends, and it was clear she was someone people wanted to be around.

I was traveling here and there, chasing jobs, but Peggy kept finding more work that needed doing—and since it gave me a reason to keep showing up, I didn't mind. Then, things between us just fell into place. Unbeknownst to me, part of fate's behind-the-scenes work would take place at a birthday party I threw on October 25, 1992. I invited a big crowd and made sure Peggy knew about it. She showed up with a plate of homemade cookies, foreshadowing many cookies to come, and a girlfriend as her plus one. The party went swimmingly, and at one point, Peggy's friend saw me and whispered to her, "He's cute—you should go out with him." I wish Peggy's friend had given me the memo, as men tend to be oblivious to matters of the heart.

Maybe I didn't recognize the signs that Peggy might be interested, or perhaps I had a mental block about it because she was a client. Whatever the reason, I didn't ask her out until two months later at the turn of the new year. As we grew closer, she wanted me to meet Robin Russell, one of her best friends who lived in Park City, because we were both due to be in the area at the same time. Meeting Robin gave me a window into Peggy's world, and there was something affirming about meeting her and knowing that Peggy and I shared similar circles and liked the same types of people. Something clicked, and it gave me an excuse to reach out to Peggy again.

Our first date was January 5, 1993, at Buckeye Roadhouse in Sausalito. It wasn't full of grand, sweeping romance; Peggy is grounded, straightforward, and practical to the core, so she didn't go for theatrics or overly sentimental gestures. That wasn't her style, and honestly, it wasn't mine either—in fact, she recalls me saying, "Let's have dinner to discuss the window project," with no insinuation of anything more.

While this may have been true, there was something more subtle brewing between us as we were seated at the bar counter that evening. I felt something stir in me as the noises around us faded into a gentle hum. Sitting close beside her, I reached over and rested my hand on her leg—a small gesture, but full of everything I hadn't yet said.

A few weeks later, during our first evening together at her place, I offered to make her dinner. Little did I know I was foreshadowing my future role as the family cook. My roommate at the time had offered what seemed like solid advice: "Bring a bottle of champagne, trust me—it'll set the tone. She'll love it." I arrived, bottle in hand, a bit nervous but willing to lean into the moment—but in true Peggy fashion, she took the bottle without much more than a nod and thanks and stashed it in the fridge. As we proceeded to cook and hang out that evening, she made no acknowledgment that maybe the champagne was something to be opened, shared, or used to make toasts. Perhaps she was keeping the bottle for a more special occasion?

I could almost hear my friend laughing, but it was classic Peggy. The romance, I'd come to realize, wasn't in the champagne or the gestures. It was in her company, unadorned honesty, and how she never pretended to be anything other than herself. And slowly, that was precisely what drew me in.

Our first year of courting was an oddball blend of spontaneity and fun. I think we both had to get to a point where we felt comfortable enough with each other to go from a working relationship to casually dating. Our courtship soon became marked by her leaving fresh cookies in my truck on random days; in return, I would gather wildflowers after work and surprise her with a hand-picked bouquet. We spent the year weaving in and around each other's lives, sharing moments that gradually turned from friendly dating into something more serious.

Peggy wasn't just a client or even a new girlfriend. She was someone who fit into my life in ways I hadn't fully anticipated. She was the kind of person who turned two simple remodels into a pivotal chapter of my life. Her presence felt natural, as if it were simply meant to be. Before I knew it, we were walking side-by-side with her beloved rottweiler and black lab in tow, Tosca and Zoey. These dogs were not just her loyal companions; they offered her security and provided additional sets of ears, which came in handy.

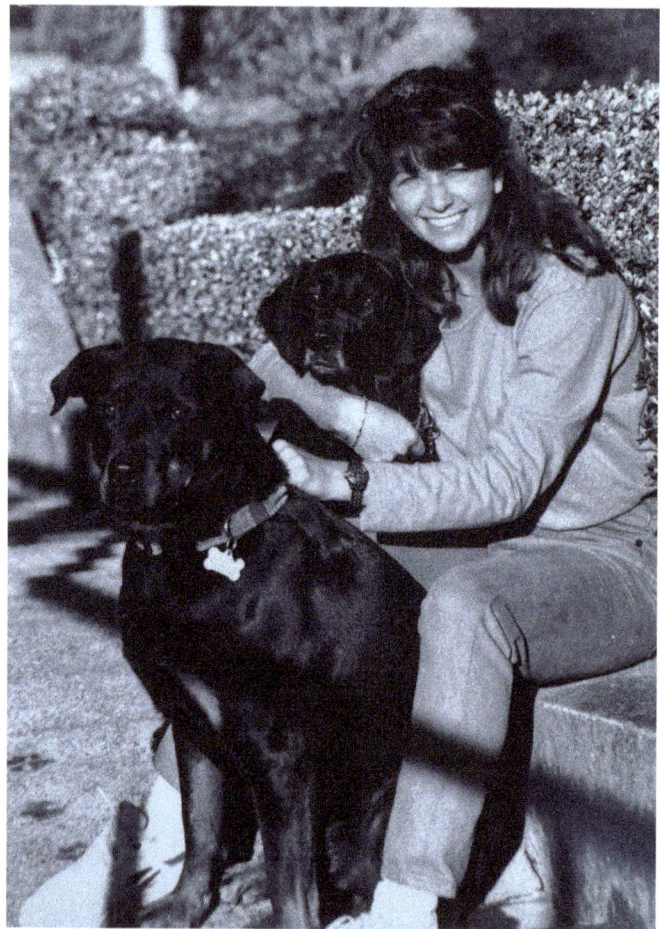

Peggy with her beloved dogs, Tosca and Zoey

It was hard not to notice Peggy's hearing aids—they were a quiet but constant presence, small devices that rarely left her ears. Early on, she told me that she and both of her brothers, Charlie and Donnie, had been born with varying degrees of hearing impairment. What struck me most wasn't Peggy's condition itself, but how naturally and confidently she moved through the world despite it. She read lips and was able to track conversations fairly well (or, I would later learn, would just fake it when she needed to). What some might have seen as a limitation, I quickly came to recognize as a kind of quiet resilience and, in many ways, a gift. Her limited hearing sometimes caused her to miss social cues, but more often, it seemed to sharpen her other senses, heightening her awareness of the world around her, making even silence hold meaning.

Over time, I stopped thinking of it as an impairment and began to see it as something more complex, even extraordinary. It gave her a depth of perception that many people with full hearing often never developed. In our relationship, she taught me to speak with more intention and listen differently, especially when I was by her side in public settings. It was just one of many things about Peggy that made me feel lucky to share her world.

By the time I wrapped up the San Francisco Plumpjack project and my second showcase home, Peggy and I had been together for just over a year, and our appetite for city life was finally beginning to wear thin. I felt the urge for simpler surroundings that aligned better with my work and my sense of adventure. Building was a passion, and I was confident I could make it work outside the hustle of San Francisco—I just hadn't expected Peggy's response when I floated the idea. With a boldness that caught me off guard, she declared, "I don't do long-distance relationships—if you're leaving, I'm coming with you." No debate, no hesitation.

Peggy and I had hiked and biked while traveling together in Utah the summer before, so I already knew we traveled well together. So, in May 1994, we packed up my pickup truck with as much as it could hold, along with Tosca and Zoey, and hit the road, with Park City, Utah, as our first stop. There was no ring on her finger. I had spoken no promises aloud. We were two best friends leaping into a new adventure together, fully aware of the risks.

I can't say for certain her father approved, but he did once say to Peggy, "I just want to make sure you're having fun." I'm not entirely sure how much he knew about our relationship at that point, or exactly how much fun we were having, but what mattered was that she was ready to take the chance, and so was I. Mountain towns were booming, and I saw a future for my business there among them.

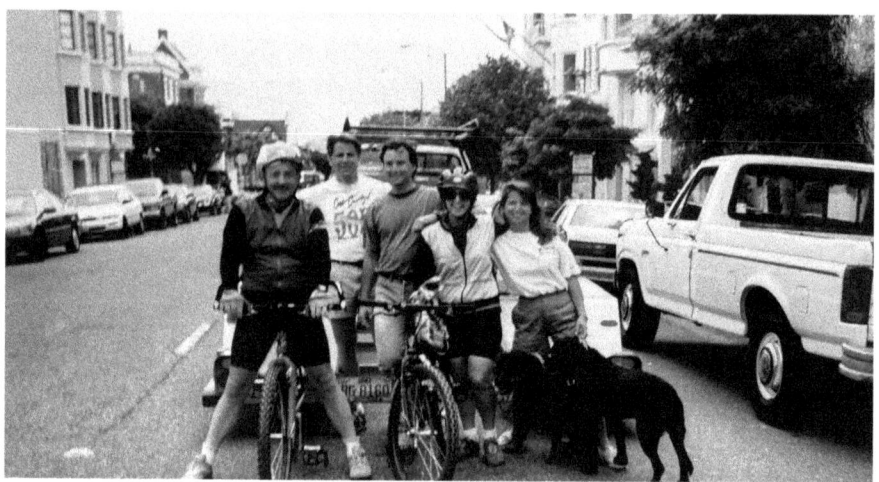
Parents and good friend Robert Tuller came by Peggy's apartment for the send-off, 1994

That summer, Peggy and I stayed in the Park City house while I helped my workmate, Mike Coakley, frame a custom home down the street. When not working, our free time was filled with adventurous bike rides and hikes through mountain trails with Tosca and Zoey. The dogs that once slept on her bed in San Francisco before we met were now sleeping outside in a makeshift shed in the yard. Thinking back, I don't believe I was showing kindness to her most important companions; it was more a reflection of my own upbringing, where our dog was loved but never lived quite so close.

Over time, I came to understand just how much she loved those two—not just as pets, but as constants in her life long before I showed up. Their quiet loyalty, and Peggy's fierce devotion to them, taught me something about love that doesn't always announce itself. I suppose their agreed-upon relocation outside was a quiet sign that I was slowly being folded into her world, but not without some negotiation. There was a dynamic forming, unspoken, where the three of us were learning how to share space in her heart.

The mountains, the excitement, the welcoming lifestyle—it all felt like home in a way San Francisco couldn't. There was no crime or gridlocked traffic. We lived in a community of people who loved being outside, breathing the same mountain air. It was a dream of a newly prioritized lifestyle that was starting to unfold.

By the late fall of 1994, as the leaves turned and snow loomed, we packed up again. This time, we were headed to my dream mountain town destination: Crested Butte, Colorado. It's hard to describe Crested Butte without sounding like a tourist brochure. There's a quiet magic there—the jagged peaks, the historic main street, the sense of a world paused in time. It's a quintessential mountain town with no chain restaurants or stores, and we fell in love with the place almost immediately. Soon, we bought our first house (more like a rustic cabin) there together.

That winter, I took on an extensive remodel of our new place. Peggy proved, yet again, to be as committed as I was, always up for an adventure should I propose one. We lived through the upheaval, sleeping under tarps and next to temporary posts holding up the floors while snow piled up outside. With a wood-burning stove as the main heat source, rising up through vents from the ground floor, she endured my half-built dreams without complaint. For all the early mornings and long days, for all the dust and the drafts, Peggy stayed by my side, even taking on projects like staining the newly hung wood siding on our home. That winter, in that unfinished house, I realized I'd found a partner willing to weather anything with me.

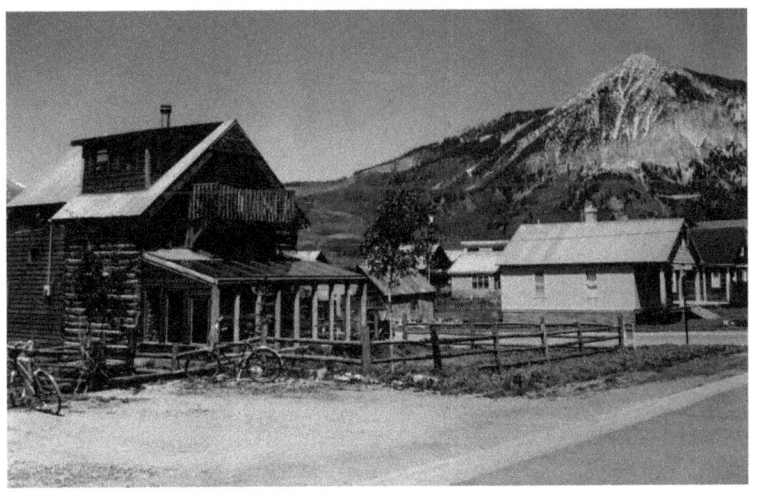

Our Crested Butte cabin, 1994

17

Tin Cup (The Town, Not the Movie)

Definition of happiness: Reality minus expectations.
—Anonymous

My life choices haven't always made sense to my parents. Even though they denied it, I'm sure they wondered if I'd lost my mind when I ran off to be a ski instructor in Jackson Hole. My mother and father also rightly questioned the wisdom of buying a house with a woman I wasn't married to. That felt risky to them. Peggy's brother, on the other hand, said that the house would hold us together more than a marriage itself.

Peggy had already been dropping hints that she wanted to get hitched—and why shouldn't we be married? She was the person I wanted to do life with. If there was an opportunity for adventure, I wanted her with me. If I snored too loud, I wanted her to be the one to pull on the sheets and tell me to turn over. Yes, it was high time we made it official, and I had the perfect plan.

It was January 14, 1995, and we were in the middle of a breathtaking dog-sledding adventure, gliding through the snowy Colorado mountains. Our destination was Tin Cup, Colorado, an old mining town that had seen its heyday long before our time. Tin Cup was basically a ghost town, visited by summer cabin dwellers and a few hearty souls who might have been staying year-round. Tin Cup had the perfect, timeless kind of silence. The bare, snow-covered streets seemed to honor those hardworking souls who once lived there.

Heart of the Journey

A few weeks earlier, I had told my parents I was planning to propose. I already had an engagement ring in hand, and they were thrilled I was finally ready to settle down. They offered diamonds from my grandmother's brooch, which we later had set into a ring from Peggy's mother, customized to hold those stones. Merging two family heirlooms into one ring felt like the perfect symbol of our bond. There was just one hurdle left before I could pop the question.

I felt traditionally bound to ask Peggy's father, Jim, if I had his permission to marry his daughter. Jim was the formidable figurehead of a successful business who had strong opinions. I knew he might have reservations about his daughter gallivanting through the Colorado wilderness with a guy who wanted to ask for her hand in marriage. Added to that, I'd only met Jim once.

Earlier in 1994, Jim came for a visit. In the eleven years Peggy had lived out West, it was the first time he'd made the trip—partly for business. We had tagged along to a dinner he'd set up with one of his vendors, and it went well. I hit it off with Peggy's stepmom, Vicki, but I couldn't get a good read on Jim throughout the evening. He seemed more intent on catering to his client than getting to know me. That's not to say our interaction was bad—just about as good as it gets when you're dating someone's daughter.

I told myself there would be plenty of time for conversation the longer I dated his daughter, but there really wasn't—he wasn't the type to reach out or engage in any small talk. The only reason I knew he was still around was because of his weekly call with Peggy. This phone call I was about to make would be the only time we had ever spoken man-to-man.

I wasn't scared to ask Jim for Peggy's hand, but I wish I'd been able to ask her mom, Dorothy, instead. Dorothy and I got along famously from the first time we met. I had the distinct feeling that as long as Peggy was happy, that was truly all that mattered to her mom. She even took to calling me "Saint John." I'm not sure where that came from, but you don't question anything that the mother of the woman you love wants to call you. Her mom was also a golfer. I wasn't a great golfer at the time, but I still played with her whenever possible. Needless to say, I would have much rather asked Dorothy for Peggy's hand.

John Baker

***

My daughter Blair once said, "My dad's parents are more normal, but my mom's parents are more fun!" Peggy's family was the one with all the color and chaos, the kind that makes for far better stories.

I'm not certain I've ever met anyone like Peggy (a nickname for Margaret). I actually find it endearing when some of her oldest friends in Sun Valley call her Margaret instead of Peggy.

She spent her early years at 201 Apple Tree Road in Winnetka, Illinois—a childhood far removed from mine in the city of San Francisco. Her parents divorced when she was just seven, and from then on, she and her two brothers lived with their mother, visiting their father on Sundays for dinners that were anything but ordinary.

Peggy fondly recalls how her father would invent quirky challenges for the kids, often around the dinner table: memorizing Roman numerals, reciting the names of U.S. presidents in order, or writing short stories—all with the promise of a silver dollar as reward. If their rooms were messy, he wouldn't scold; instead, he'd dump the contents of their drawers on the floor with theatrical flair and declare, "Now, let's clean up your room." There were also legendary family Monopoly matches that added to the fabric of growing up in the Mills house. The games and contests were training grounds for grit, humor, and perspective.

To understand Peggy, you really have to understand her father, who was brilliant, eccentric, and a firm believer in turning life on its head. Jim had a reputation for being difficult at times with his kids. He could be hard, direct, even unyielding, but he was also a sharp and insightful man with a knack for cutting to the point and getting things done. In his own way, Jim could be enlightening. He had a kind of blunt wisdom and wasn't afraid to share it, usually with a few choice words. He was a man who knew what he wanted, even if that meant coming across a bit direct, unfiltered, and, at rare times, even unintentionally funny.

I've always found myself drawn to people who excel in certain areas of life yet fall short in others—those who, while flawed, have a kind of brilliance that can't be ignored. I'm not talking about failures of character or morality. I mean people who sometimes struggle socially, who might be hard to get along with or even considered prickly. These same people can be exceptional in other realms, and I tend to feel compassion for them. They're good human beings in their own right, just complicated ones. That was Jim.

Peggy's father remarried soon after the divorce, blending in two stepsisters, Deidre and Margueritte. Peggy, ever adaptable, embraced the new dynamic and learned to navigate two households with a certain self-made freedom. That independence blossomed further in high school, when her best friend Diana—whose father owned Park West, a nightclub in downtown Chicago—introduced her to an entirely new world. Still underage, the two of them would sneak into Park West on Saturday nights, soaking in the buzz of the city and the music; Peggy would always have her hair worn long, to hide the hearing aids she was still shy about.

Peggy left Chicago when she was eighteen to go to UC San Diego. Then, after graduating, she found her way to San Francisco. While the formative years with her family in Chicago shaped her as a person, she's really been out West most of her life. Like her father, Peggy has continued to place the importance of family at the top of her list. She still cherishes family dinner and sees it as a time to get everyone around the table. The irony is that she doesn't have the patience for late reservations or long dinners, so it's really an excuse to round everyone up and check in on her terms. If you want to eat dinner, then you better plan your day around that meal. At home, I'm cooking; in Hawaii or during other travels, we're out somewhere nice. You can be gone all day—but you'd better not be late to that dinner reservation.

***

After clearing my pop psychology thoughts, I prepared to make the call. I waited until Peggy went outside to walk the dogs and composed myself as I dialed Jim's direct office number.

The phone rang, and someone picked it up. "Hello," a voice answered briskly, sounding like Jim's younger brother, Jon Mills.

"Jon?" I asked, trying to keep my nerves from showing.

"Yes," came the reply.

"Oh. Hi, Jon. It's John Baker, actually trying to reach Jim."

"Is everything all right? Is there anything we can do?"

I chuckled, my anxiety simmering under my casual tone. "Well, yes, we're fine. There's nothing we need at this time, just trying to reach Jim. Can you connect me?"

"Yes, hold on a sec. You sure there's nothing we can do for you?" he asked, sounding concerned.

"Nothing at all," I replied, laughing a bit. "We're just out here enjoying Crested Butte."

"I'll transfer you," said Jon.

A moment later, the phone clicked over. "This is Jim," he said, his voice curt and direct.

"Hi, Jim. It's John. Peggy's boyfriend."

"Hi, John," he said in a flat tone that didn't give much away. This was it.

"Well, I ... I was calling to ask if I can marry your daughter," I stammered.

There was a pause, one that stretched just long enough for doubt to rush in. Then, in his blunt, straightforward way, he asked, "Why are you asking me?"

I swallowed hard, my heart dropped. For a second, I thought I'd completely blown it. His question caught me off guard. Was this a test, or just Jim being Jim? After a brief pause to collect myself, I replied, "Since you raised her, and I want to spend the rest of my life with her, I wanted to ask for your permission."

"Okay," he said finally, his tone softening. "That's fine. Vicki and I would like to do whatever we can for the two of you and wish you the best lives together."

Before I could even fully process it, the line clicked. Peggy's dad was gone. I don't know what else I expected. I didn't think he was going to offer me a dowry or ask for my last three tax returns. I allowed myself to be relieved, if not a bit shaken. I hung up the phone and took a deep breath. I had his blessing. Now, all I needed was to ask Peggy. Thankfully, I had a better plan for that than I'd had for speaking with her father.

Heart of the Journey

When Peggy got back in from dog walking, we made plans for the day's group sled trip. Somehow, I contained myself as the sled dogs were hooked to the harness and then to the sled. The dogs were excited and barking, but that seemed normal—maybe it was all genetic memory for them, or they genuinely loved to run. Whatever the reason, they couldn't wait to get moving, and when we were all set, the musher gave a command, and we took off. There was an exhilarating surge of power and speed as the dogs lunged forward in perfect harmony. Snow sprayed all around as the dogs' feet kicked up the fine powder. The sled itself felt like it had come to life in a smooth, thrilling glide down the trail.

The mountains rose around us as the dogs pulled us ever forward. Like a switch had been flipped, I felt ready to ask my question—I had already made up my mind before, but now I felt at perfect peace with my decision. I felt serenity with the cold air hitting my face and Peggy in my arms, the dogs' panting and the crunch of snow underneath the sled the only sounds in the world around us.

At the run's halfway point, we stopped in the town of Tin Cup to rest the dogs. That would give us a chance to walk around the old buildings and explore a bit before heading back. In a moment when Peggy wasn't paying attention, I slipped the ring into my jacket pocket. Then I said, "Let's go check out that old schoolhouse." We made our way through the deep snowfield. When we got closer to the building, I paused and took a moment to look around. I wanted to savor the moment and remember it forever.

The quiet, the snow, the crisp mountain air—all of it created a sense of timelessness that felt just right. I reached into my pocket and started to pull out the ring. I took a breath, preparing to get down on one knee. But just as I was about to open my mouth, Peggy announced, "I need to pee."

At first, I couldn't process what she'd said. It made more sense when she turned away from me and dropped her pants. Then, she did what nature called her to do. I couldn't help but laugh to myself. First, there was her dad's curveball, and now this. It was like Peggy and her father had some telepathic connection and were hell-bent on throwing me off my game. One thing was for sure: The romantic, picture-perfect proposal I'd envisioned was gone.

I'd never get that moment back again, but my Hallmark card moment was replaced by something infinitely more real. When you forge a life with someone, maybe 1 percent of your time together is suitable for framing and putting on the living room wall. The other 99 percent is just authentically real. In its own way, Peggy's call of the wild made this moment even more perfect—because it was real, and that was us.

When she finished, I didn't wait for another chance to kneel. Instead, I ran over and playfully embraced her, both of us falling into the deep snow, my face just inches from hers. I kissed her, then asked, "Will you marry me?"

"Are you serious?" she replied.

"I am."

"Really?"

We stood up, and I could see she was so happy—but that thought was interrupted when I realized she still hadn't answered.

"You still haven't said yes!" I said.

It was a bit of a blur, but finally, Peggy said, "Yes!"

"I have a ring," I replied, sliding it onto her finger, the golden band somehow making it official in my mind.

We marched back through the snow holding hands, greeted by the other dog sledders. When we got back, we shared the bottle of champagne I had stashed away.

Life, I realized, isn't a perfect photograph. It's a collection of imperfect, unforgettable moments, stitched together by shared trust, laughter, challenges. It's choosing each other, again and again. And if you're lucky, you get to stumble through it all with someone who turns even the most unceremonious pee break into part of the love story.

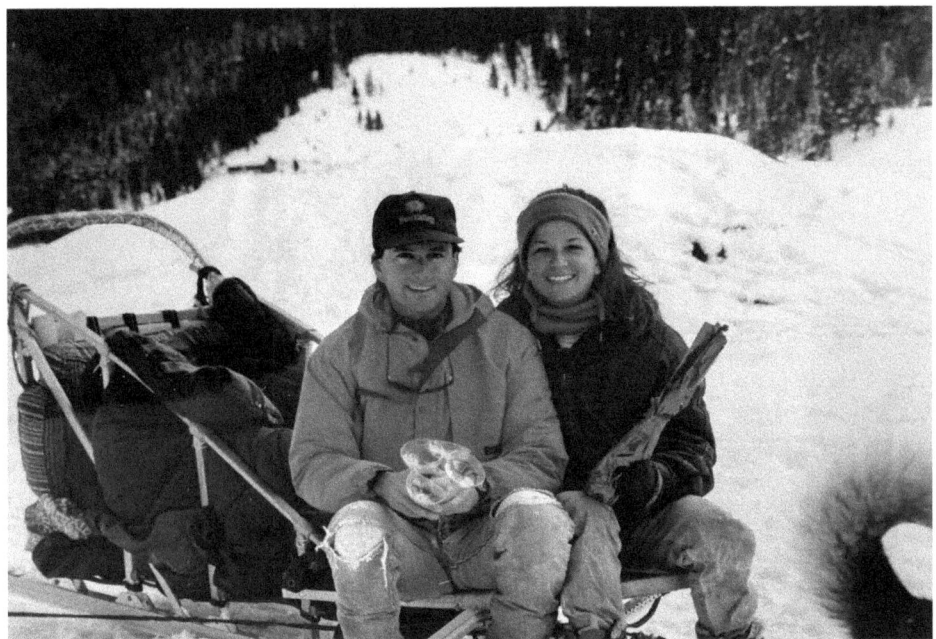

Tin Cup proposal, January 14, 1995

When I told my parents that Peggy and I were engaged later that afternoon, they didn't offer advice or judgment. They simply responded with heartfelt joy, welcoming another daughter-in-law into the family with open arms. That was their quiet gift: unwavering support, no matter where the road led. My parents might not have understood every decision I made—the ski bum detour, the house before the vows, the unconventional path—but they never withheld their confidence in me.

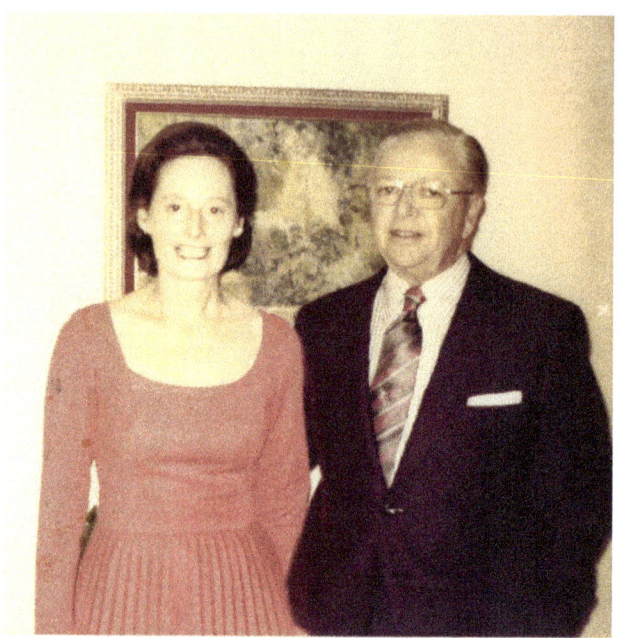

My grandparents, Theresa (Terry) and Stan Breyer, 1973

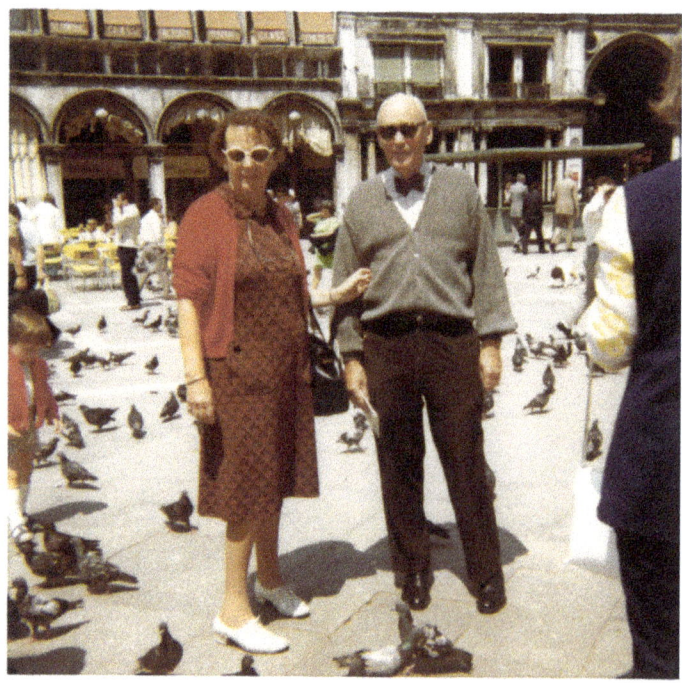

Virginia and Harry Baker, Venice, Italy

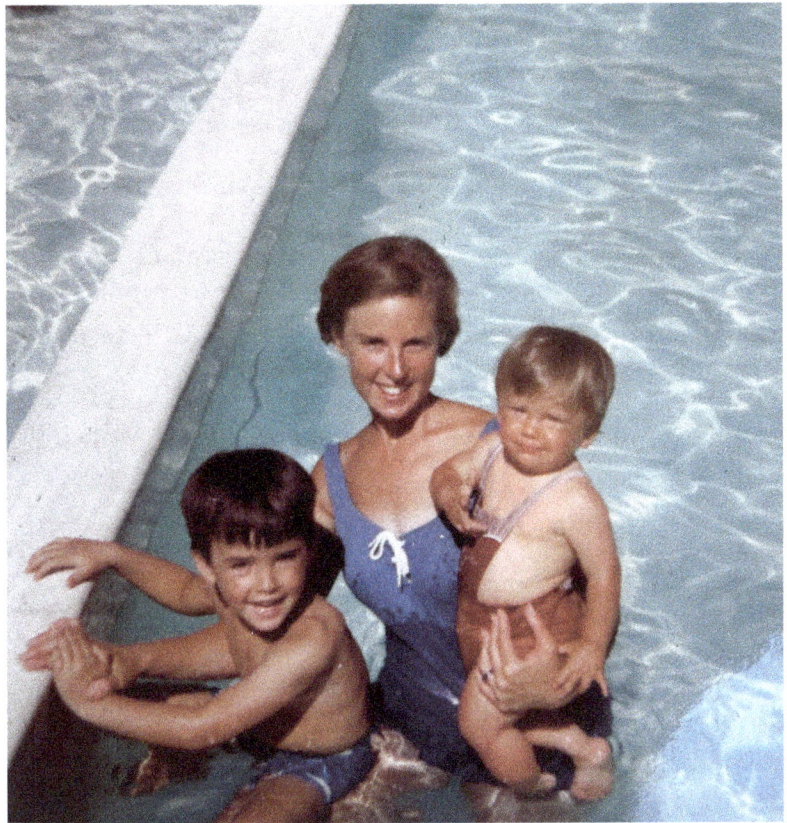
Tahoe Tavern with mom and brother Chris, 1968

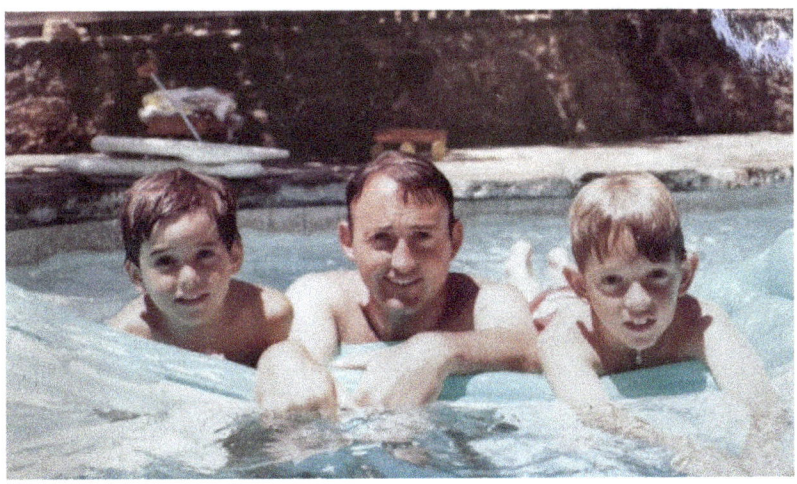
Kentfield with my father and brother Wayne, July 1969

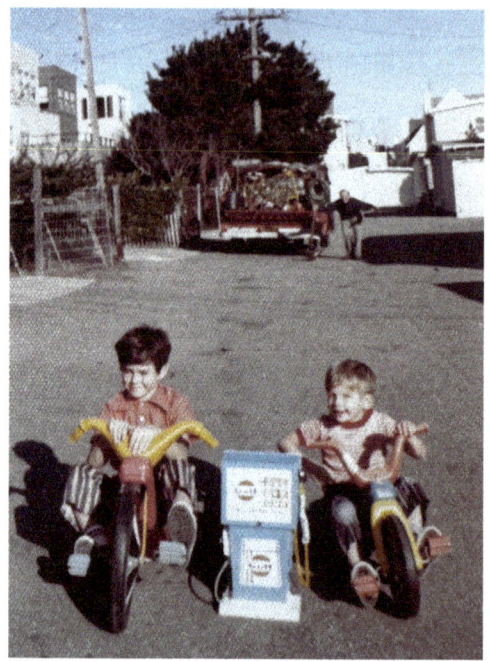

Me and my brother Chris on Big Wheels in the alley

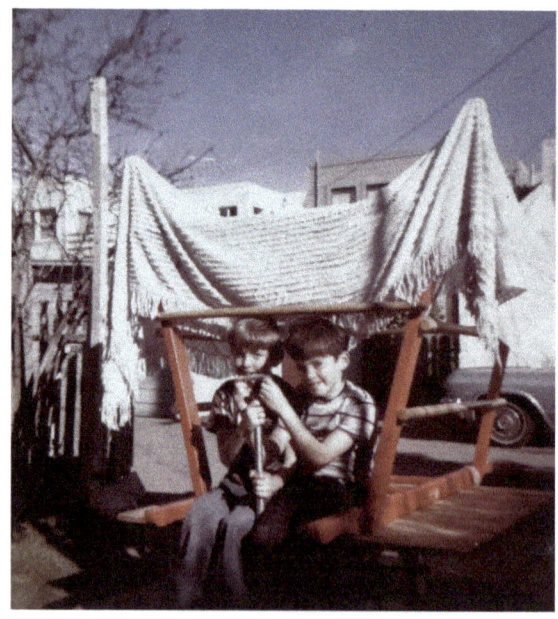

Alley on 29th Ave—makeshift covered wagon with my brother Wayne

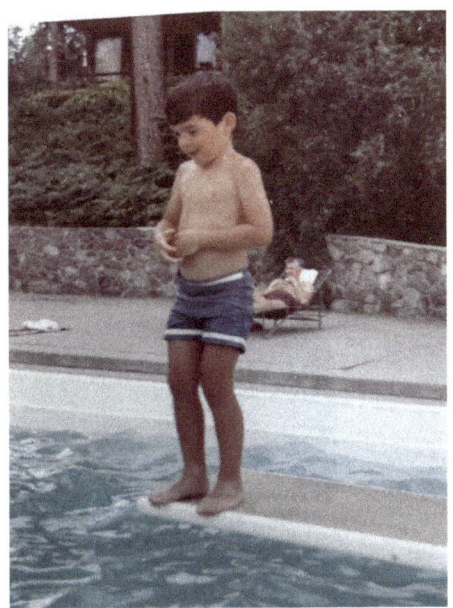
Timid on the diving board above the deep end

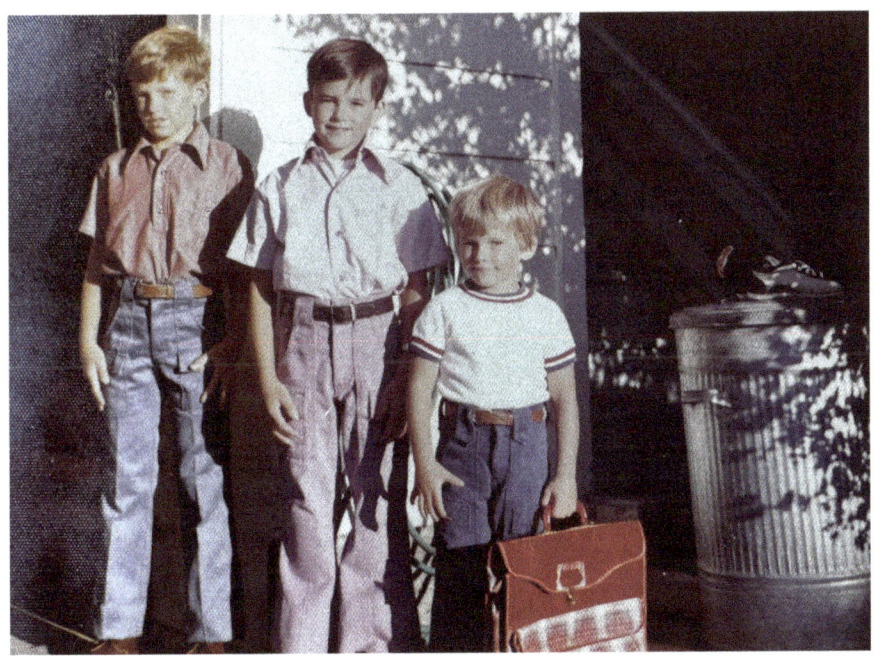
First day of school with brothers Wayne and Chris, 1972

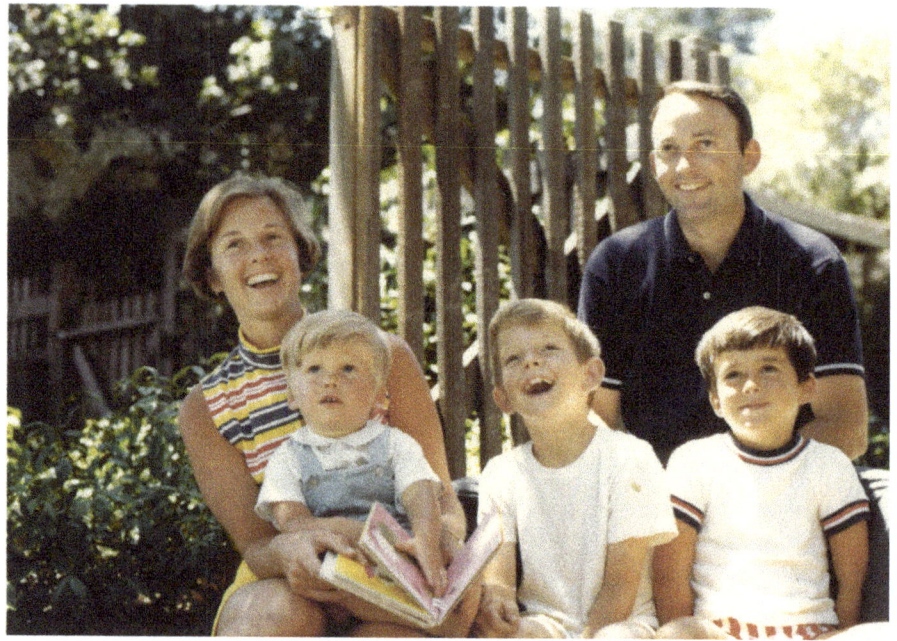
Making fond memories at our grandparents' place in Kent Woodlands

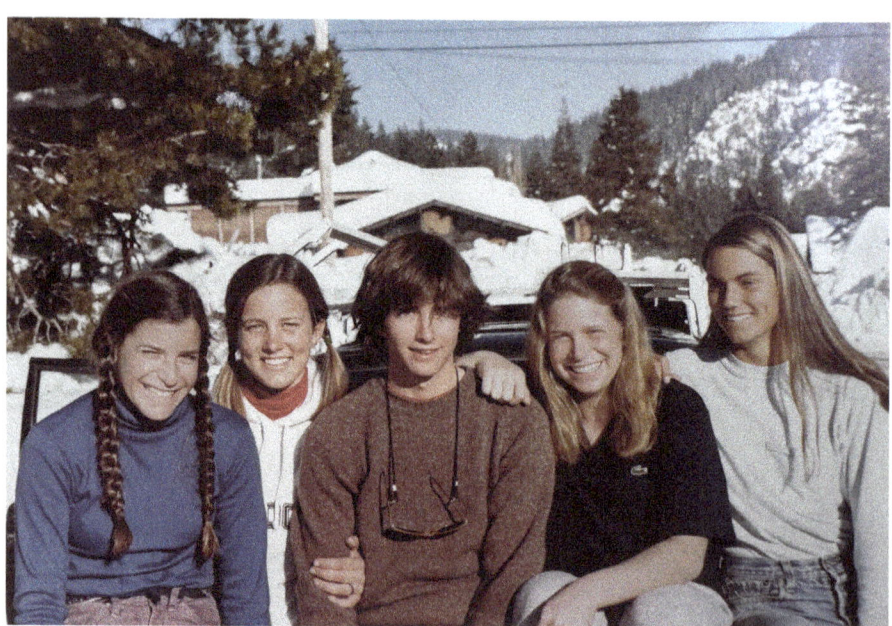
High school was a cool time

Heart of the Journey

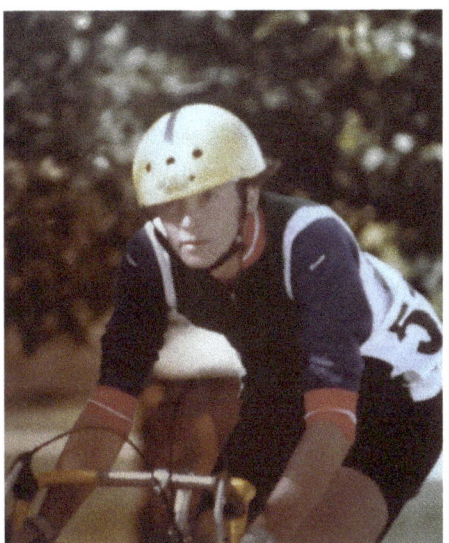

Road race in Boulder, Colorado

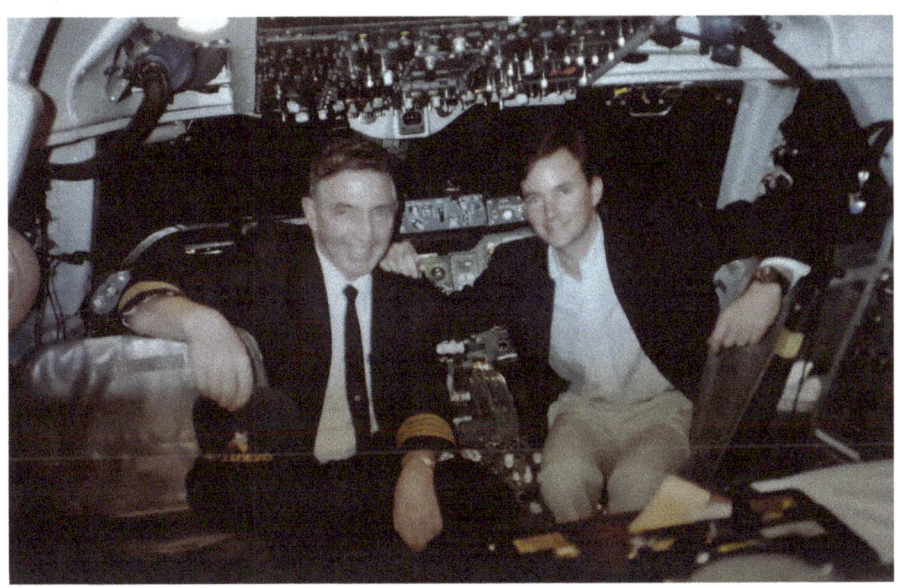

Me with my godfather, John Bell, a 747 Captain

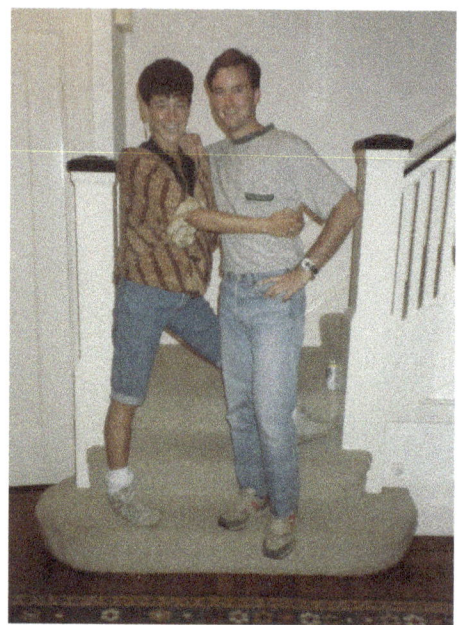

Reunion with next door neighbor, Renee Goddard

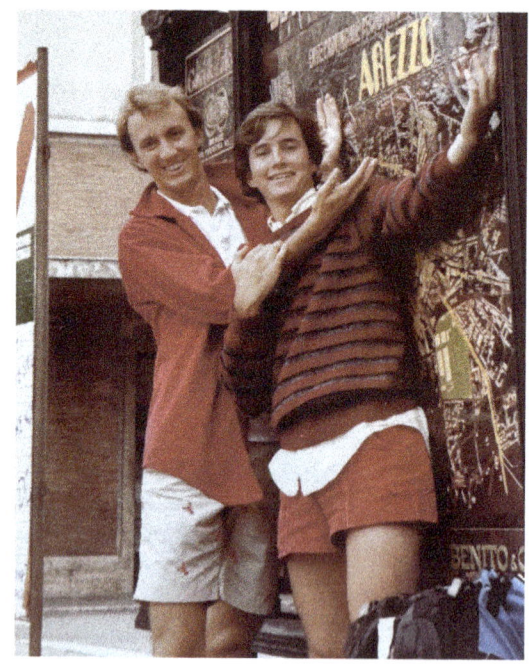

Traveling with Beau in Arrezzo, Italy, 1983

Heart of the Journey

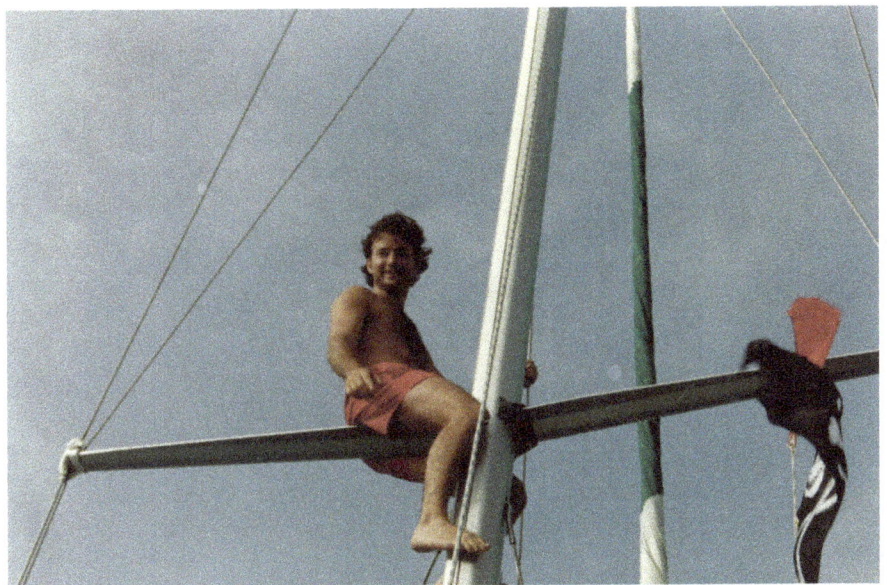

British Virgin Islands, 1988

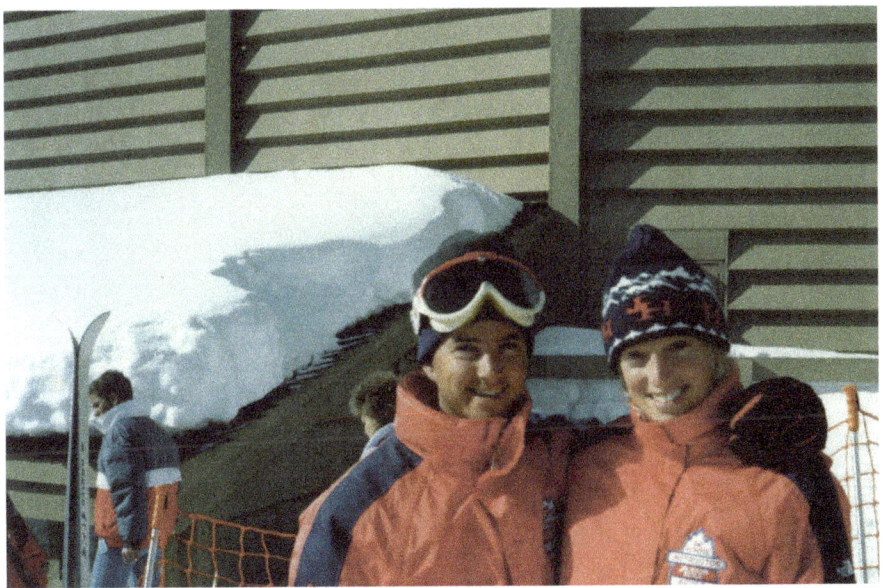

Jackson Hole Ski School uniforms with Katie Knick, Winter 1988

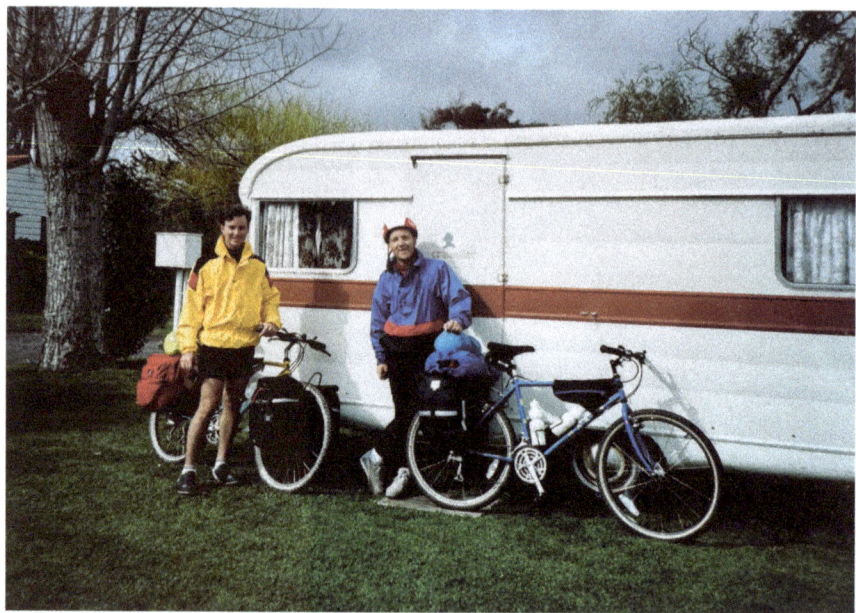
New Zealand accommodations with Griff Towle, 1989

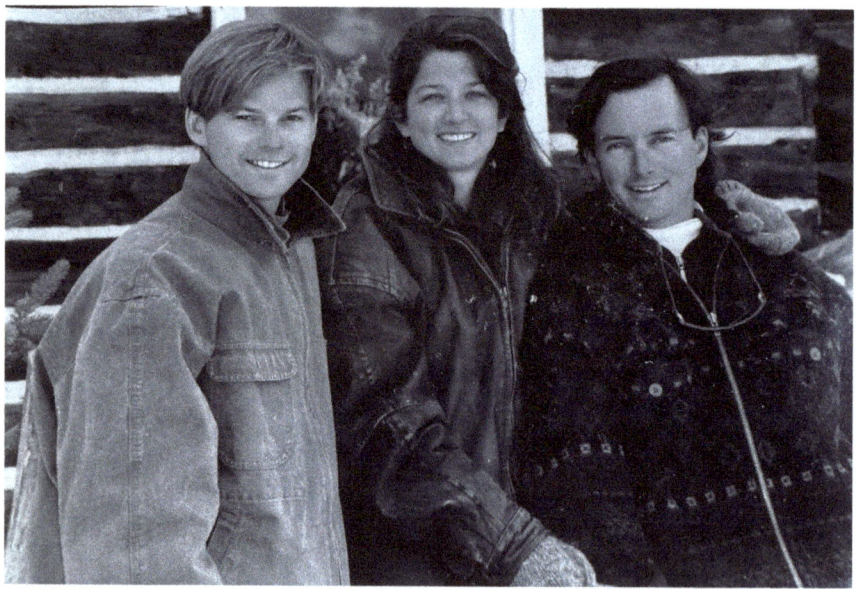
Winter in Crested Butte with Peggy and brother Chris, 1994

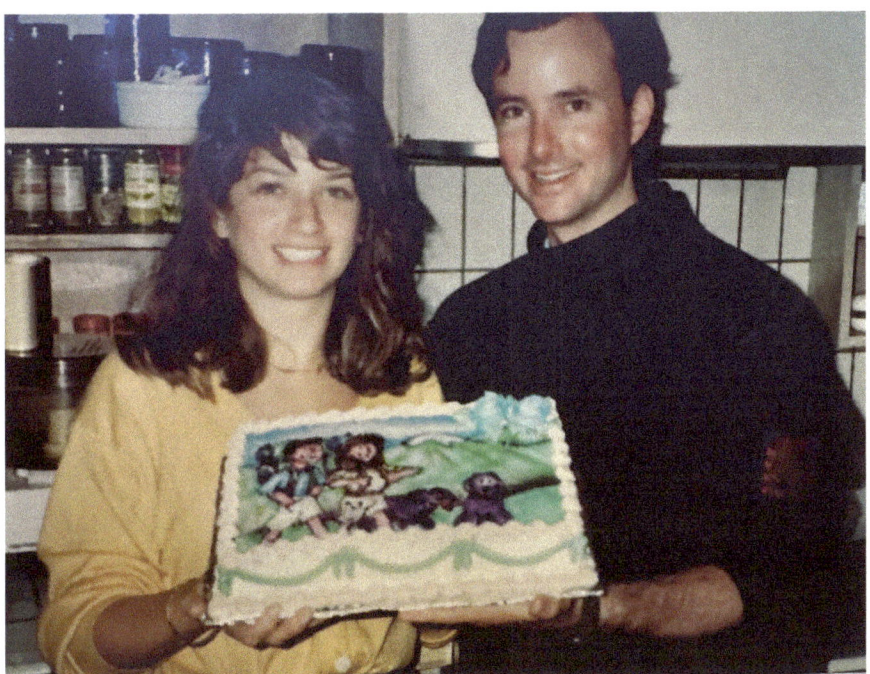

Courting days, 1993

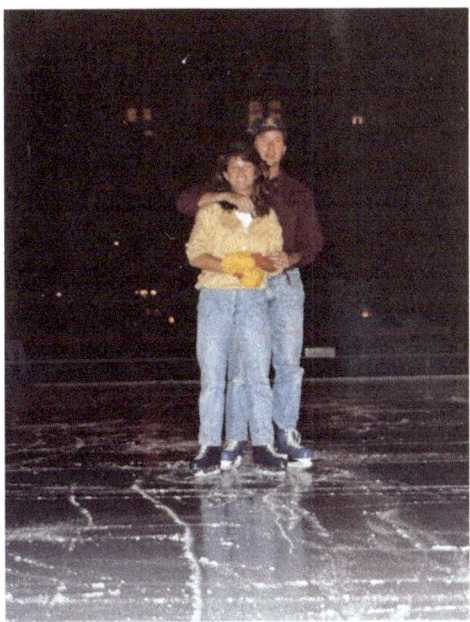

Visiting Sun Valley on a road trip, 1993

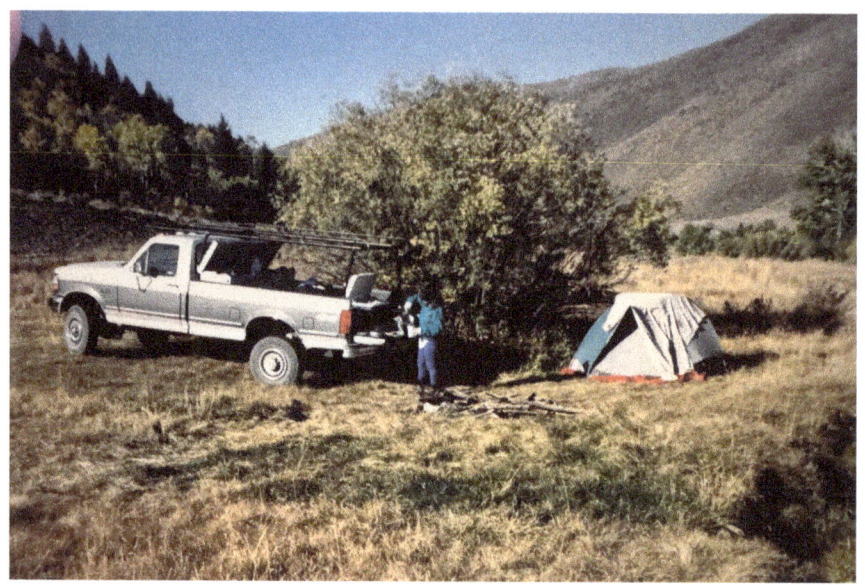

First time together in Sun Valley, camping out at Corral Creek, 1993

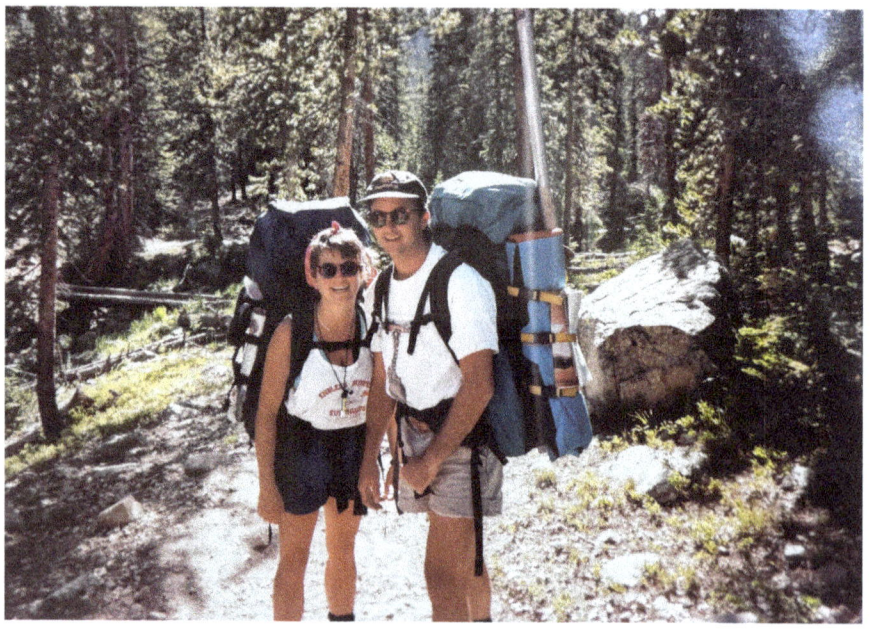

Backpacking in the early days

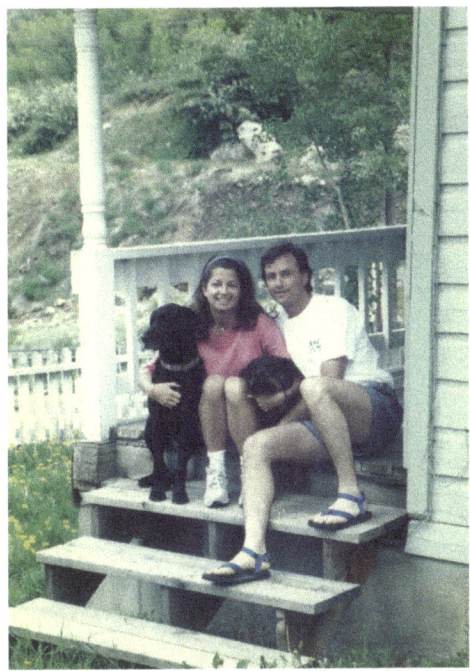

Park City house, Summer 1994

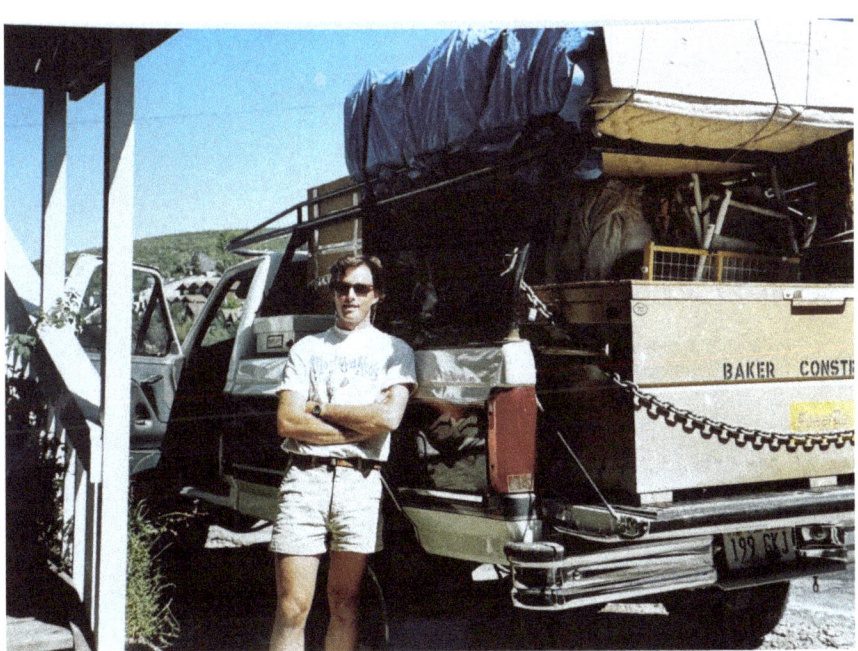

Packed up and heading to Crested Butte, Colorado, 1994

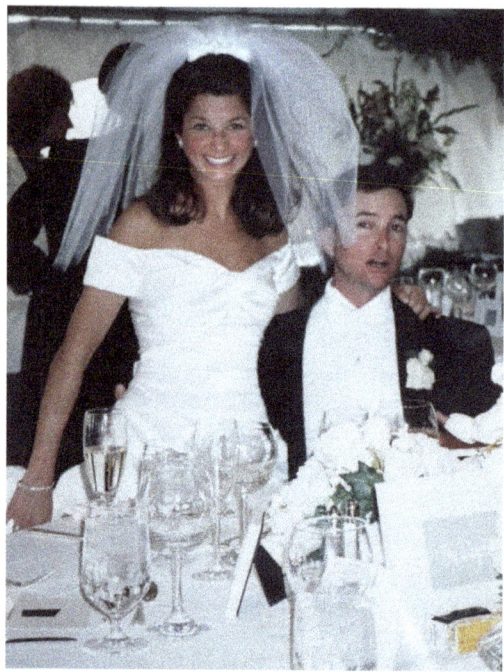

Wedding on June 3, 1995

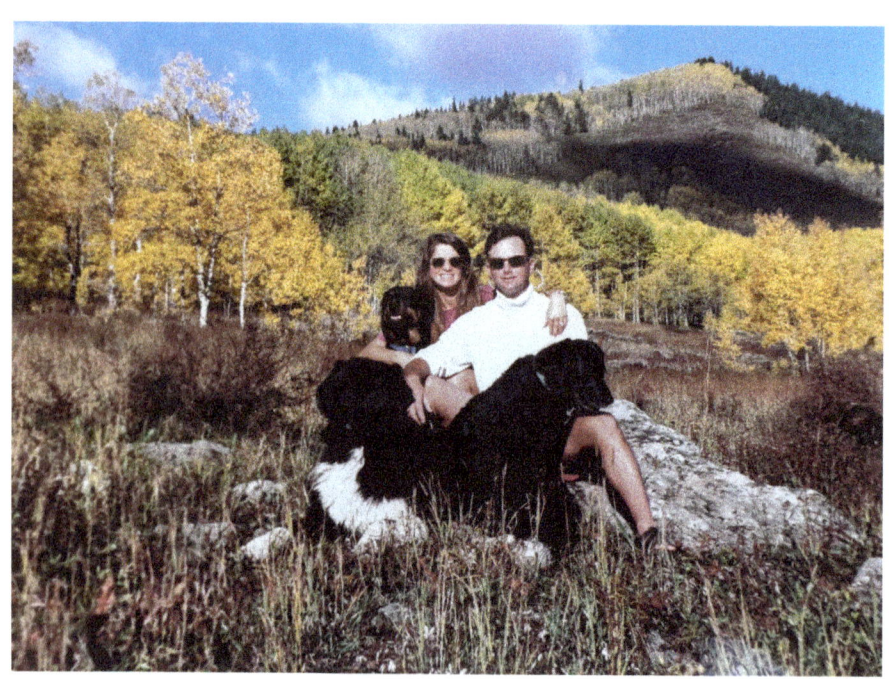

In Crested Butte, Fall 1996 with Tosca, Zoey, and Bradley

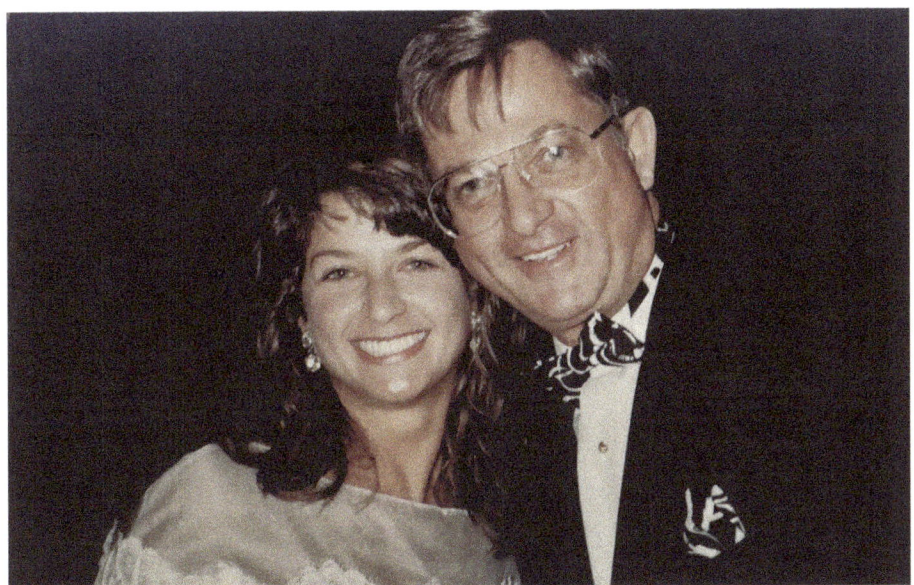
Peggy with her father, Jim Mills

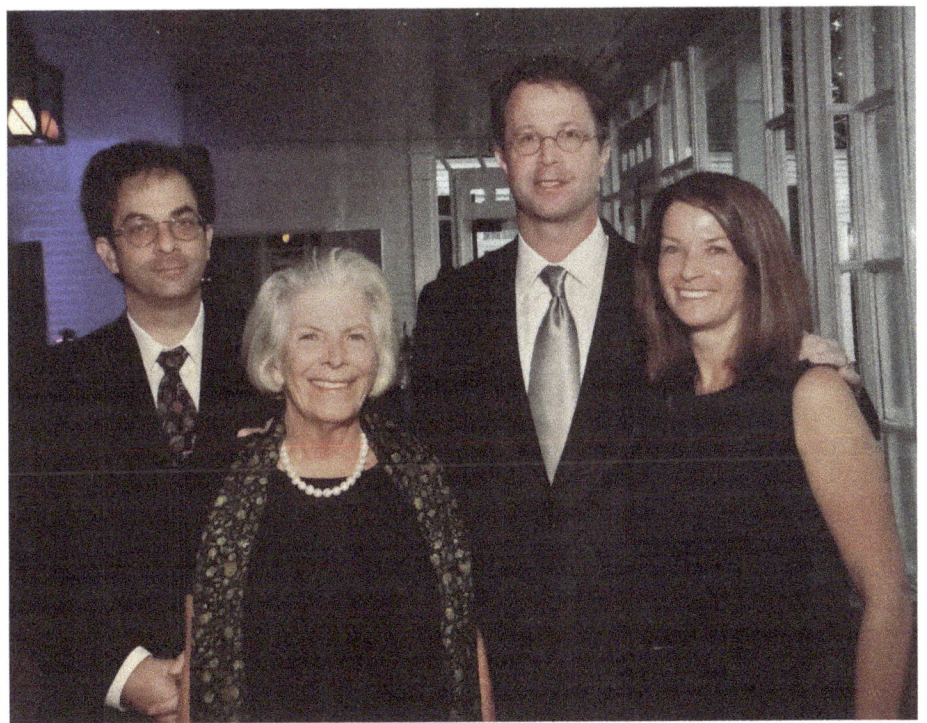
Donnie, Charlie, and Peggy Mills, with their mother, Dorothy

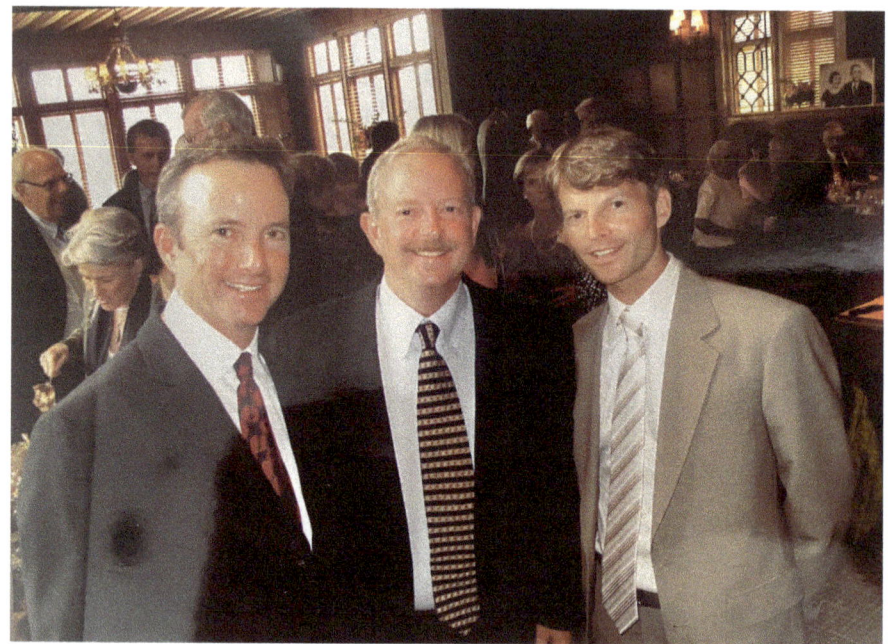

Brothers Wayne and Chris at our parents' 50th wedding anniversary, September 13, 2009

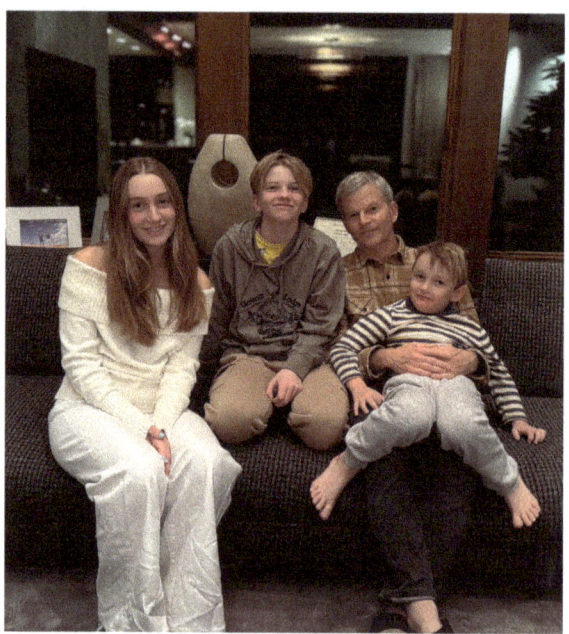

Brother Chris and his children Sadie, Alice, and Sasha

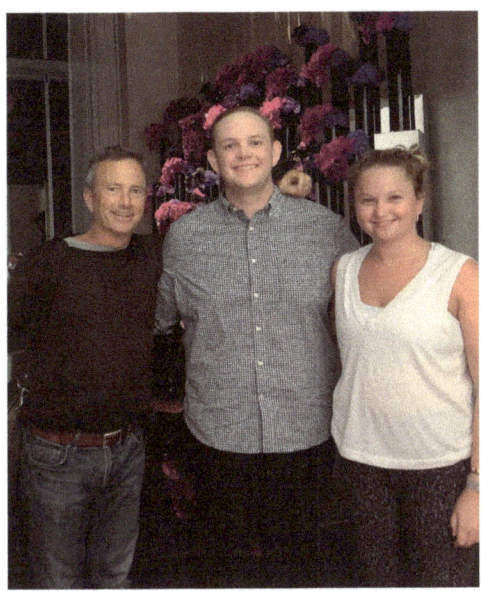

Nephew Harry Baker with Blair and me

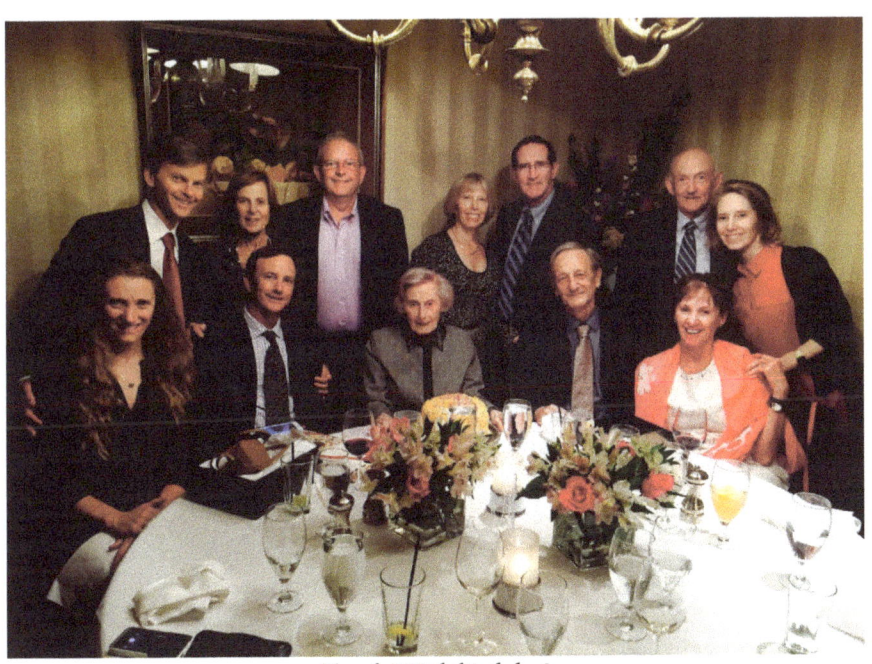

Terry's 100th birthday!

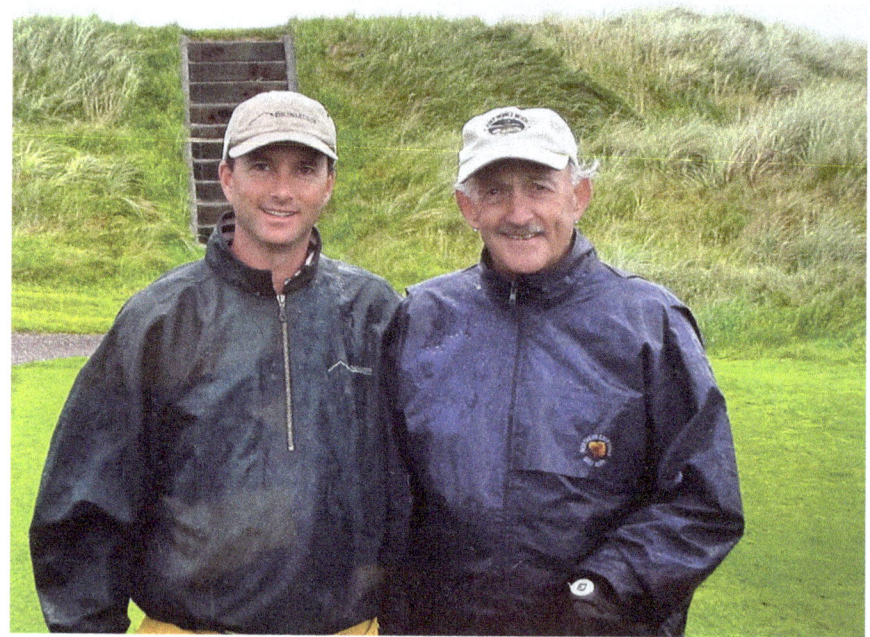

World Father and Son Golf Tournament, Waterville, Ireland, 2003

18

Avalanche

*We should certainly count our blessings,
but we should also make our blessings count.*
—Neal A. Maxwell

During the early winter months of 1995, I was working with a contractor, helping him build a house in a secluded neighborhood up Coal Creek Canyon, outside Crested Butte. The journey to the jobsite took me through a narrow canyon notorious for avalanches in winter, a fact everyone who ventured there knew well. The danger started high up in a place called Red Lady Bowl. At the top of the bowl, snow accumulated. The freeze-thaw cycle frequently created dangerous slide conditions, sending destructive avalanches roaring down the canyon.

The locals took the threat seriously. In fact, the road that ran through the canyon had stark signs posted along the route: No Stopping—Avalanche Area. These weren't deer crossing signs that you quickly forgot after seeing; anyone who drove up Coal Creek in midwinter understood that just passing through that area meant putting your life on the line. But one morning, in late February of 1995, I carelessly broke the rule.

Snow was coming down so thick that I couldn't see through the windshield of my Ford pickup truck. With zero visibility, I pulled over to clear the snow from the windshield, not exactly certain if I was within the avalanche zone or not—it seemed like the responsible thing to do at the time. I had lost all vision through the windshield, and poking my head out the driver's side window was problematic. It was either run the risk of an avalanche occurring at that moment or drive off a cliff. At that moment, stopping felt like my only option.

After the snow was temporarily cleared from my windshield, I got back in the cab and carefully pulled away only to notice the No Stopping—Avalanche Area signs off to one side, mostly obscured by the wind-driven snow. I drove down through a gully and up to the jobsite without another thought. When I arrived just a few minutes later, I had no idea what had just transpired. Suddenly, a man pulled up on a snowmobile and asked me a question that froze me in my tracks: "Is everyone on your team accounted for?"

I looked at him confused and asked, "Why?"

He pointed back toward the road below. "Red Lady Bowl just slid. The whole area you just passed through is buried. Forty to fifty feet of snow, ice, and debris came down and wiped out the gully and all in its path."

I felt a chill, but my shiver wasn't from the below-freezing temperatures. My visceral reaction was that I wouldn't have been standing there if I had been pulled over for just a minute longer. To put it bluntly, Peggy almost lost me just before our wedding.

In the days after the avalanche, I replayed the scenario in my mind countless times. I'd lie awake at night, wondering what I could have done differently. Those few moments and the solitary decision to pull over ran through my mind like I was watching the instant replay of a fourth down in a football game. I was having an existential crisis: My life had been spared, but why? I didn't know how long it had been after I drove off that the avalanche hit. Was it three minutes? Had I escaped death by only thirty seconds? What if I'd driven a little faster or slower that day? What force aligned the moon and stars enough that I escaped a fate I didn't know was a possibility?

When I tell this story today, my daughter Blair likes to remind me of the "burnt toast" theory—the metaphorical concept that suggests small, seemingly negative events can lead to positive outcomes. It derives from the idea that if you burn your toast in the morning and have to remake it, you might spark a chain reaction of delays that prevent you from being in the wrong place at the wrong time later in the day.

The avalanche was a close call, closer than I'd like to admit. Sure, I'd had a few brushes with getting hurt skiing, road riding, or daredevil high-speed mountain biking, but surviving those incidents was easily explained away as my superior skills keeping me safe. That was a young man's game, covering mortality with a fresh layer of bullshit—though why shouldn't the young feel invincible? It wasn't until we got older and saw the plate of horrors life could dish out that we understood just how many things were coming at us. I'd always pushed the boundaries, often putting myself in situations that, in hindsight, might've seemed reckless. Right or wrong, I now see that I did those things either to prove my skills or to conquer my fears.

The avalanche experience shook me, but it didn't keep me from taking risks. There's a certain confidence, or maybe arrogance, that comes with feeling like you can handle whatever life throws your way. This holds true in all other aspects of life as well. The more you don't die, the more you feel that you can pull yourself out of tight spots with nothing but grit. Those thoughts usually evaporate as you get older, have kids, or experience something so profound it leaves a lasting mark. But there was always a lingering question I should have been asking: *At what point does my luck run out or my number quietly come up?*

Any existential dread I felt from the avalanche experience faded as the winter of 1995 went on. The shift in mood was due to growing tired of constantly looking over my shoulder for threats I had conjured up in my mind.

In my later years, I was hiking in Zermatt below the Matterhorn with Peggy and watched two teenagers barreling down the mountain on bikes. There were no elbow or knee pads for these teens, who wore nothing but T-shirts, shorts, and helmets. They grinned from ear to ear, daring gravity to challenge them. I watched one of them fly off a ridge, slide out to the side, and then correct himself at the last possible second. The dust as he tore down the path made it so I could barely see the outcome. I couldn't help but think, *That was me.* That confidence, that willingness to dance on the edge—it was something I recognized immediately.

My close call in Coal Creek Canyon was only the beginning. Since then, I've faced other near-misses: rocks kicked out above me while climbing the Grand Teton, getting caught alone in a snow well under a tree while skiing off-piste, having a close call with a shark. Those were times I wondered if I had pushed my luck a little too far. There's a strange feeling that comes with surviving those moments—a kind of surreal gratitude. It was as if I'd built up a bank account of risks and close calls, and I kept making withdrawals, each one bringing me closer to zero. If cats had nine lives, how many did John Baker have? Maybe there's only so much of that kind of luck you get in a lifetime. Or perhaps it's all chance—an unexplainable twist of timing and circumstance that leaves you spared for reasons you can only wonder about. Oh, did I mention the time I went skydiving out of an airplane?

19

Crossroads

*If everyone is thinking alike,
then someone isn't thinking.*

—George S. Patton Jr.

4:00 a.m., Saturday, April 27, 2024

The cardiologist, Dr. Daniels, was between the devil and the deep blue sea. Everything in his fiber told him I'd had a heart attack, but the data from the cath lab tests showed otherwise. My organs were systematically shutting down, and there was no time left. He had to act, or the deep blue sea would exact its toll on me.

I mean that in an almost literal sense. Because my blood pressure kept dropping, the medical staff kept pumping me with massive doses of vasopressors. The medication is designed to elevate blood pressure and supply needed fluids. If I remember fluid dynamics from a long-gone physics class, the more liquid that's pumped into a closed system, the higher the pressure. That's great if you get the right amount of pressure and the fluid stays in the system, but my body was hoarding liquid like a chipmunk stockpiling acorns for the winter—and most of the excess saline was pooling around my heart and lungs.

If you've ever had a child or a heavy pet sit on your chest, you know how hard it is to breathe. If something wasn't done quickly to help my heart and lungs function correctly, I would drown on dry land.

Thankfully, Dr. Daniels is a quick thinker. While driving into the hospital a half-hour earlier, he had arranged for an operating room to be prepped with an Extracorporeal Membrane Oxygenation (ECMO) machine. Many people first heard of these machines during COVID, as they were frequently used as a life support system when a patient's body was under stress and shutting down. An ECMO provides lifesaving support by taking over the functions of the heart and lungs when they are severely compromised, allowing them to rest and recover.

Blood is drawn from the patient's body and oxygenated outside the body through a specialized machine. Once filtered, the blood is pumped back into the body, ensuring it receives the oxygen it needs while removing carbon dioxide. Think of kidney dialysis, except for carbon dioxide instead of impurities in the blood.

Since blood is being pumped by the ECMO machine into the body at a positive pressure, that can cause issues if the heart isn't pumping normally—like mine. If that pressure isn't released, the lungs can fill with fluid and fail. To compensate for that excess pressure, Dr. Daniels would run tubes up my arteries from my groin to my chest and make a small hole between the two upper chambers of my heart—the atria. Then, a balloon was to be gently dilated in the opening between the atria, a procedure called an atrial septostomy. That balloon allows doctors to release the pressure on the left side of the heart and divert it into the ECMO cannulas on the right side. After the ECMO takes over, the heart can rest and recover while the machine maintains circulation and oxygenation.

Peggy was a wreck as she waited at the hospital. Her mind had to fight off the negative thoughts and search for the positive ones. From what I know about her, when adrenaline is rushing through her veins, she becomes more hyper-focused and task-oriented than usual. It's lucky for me that her attention to detail in this altered state was focused on my condition, even though she still didn't quite understand exactly what the doctors were doing to me.

Heart of the Journey

5:00 a.m., Saturday, April 27

During my surgery, the beast of a machine was calibrated and flipped on. I was now a cyborg—a machine was handling all my heart functions. Strangely, the procedure itself took less time than watching a good movie. Time had slipped through a crack in consciousness, leaving behind only blank space, a body that was being kept alive by a machine, and what would soon be three lost days.

After surgery and recovery, they wheeled me back down to the ICU and let Peggy see me for a few minutes. The ECMO machine stood large beside my bed as I lay still in medically induced sedation. A maze of vibrantly colored tubes and wires pulsated with lifesaving energy. My scarlet blood flowed through the ECMO's clear tubing as a visual reminder of the delicate process of oxygenation and filtration happening outside my body. Close to a dozen monitors blinked steadily, echoing the rhythm of borrowed time as the machine temporarily shouldered the burden of my faltering heart.

Sunrise, Saturday Morning, April 27

Sunrise that Saturday morning was at 6:18 a.m., and well before the sun came up, Peggy started calling the family. She was alone, overwhelmed, and needed support. And the people closest to me needed to know what was happening. It took remarkable courage to walk back the reassurances she'd made to our children and my extended family not twelve hours earlier. She didn't hold any culpability for my condition worsening. Still, for our kids, Mom had said everything would be all right. Now, that assertion was up in the air.

The kids were rightfully concerned and scared. Peggy tried to sound as confident and calm as possible while her emotions ran wild inside her mind and body. Without hesitation, and with their mom's assistance, the kids arranged travel to San Francisco. Wilson and Blair would fly in later that night from Boston and New York City, respectively, and Peggy's stepsister Deidre followed. Hayden would finish some final exam studies and arrive on Tuesday.

Peggy also contacted my brother Chris, who had arrived at Lake Tahoe late the night before. Once he heard that I had taken a sideways turn, he more than likely had an extra coffee or three and got back on the road. Peggy also got back in touch with my parents. With the update, Mom and Dad coordinated with Chris and started to make their way to me.

10:00 a.m., Saturday

At the start of visiting hours, Dr. Daniels came in and exchanged pleasantries with Peggy. After the chit-chat, Dr. Daniels's voice shifted into the dry, clinical tone all doctors have.

"The first thing we did was put him on the ECMO machine. That was non-negotiable. He needed it to survive, and that's what we did. That's when we landed on the diagnosis of cardiogenic shock," Dr. Daniels explained. "John's heart was failing to pump enough blood to maintain his organs. And more specifically, we diagnosed stress cardiomyopathy. It's usually caused by extreme physical or emotional stress, which weakens the heart significantly. I'm hoping we can get him off the ECMO in a few days, but we've got to figure out the underlying condition that's causing all of this."

As if on cue, another doctor walked into my ICU room—Dr. Jennifer Ling, an infectious disease specialist. The two doctors conversed in the esoteric language of medicine, which consists of one part acronyms, one part numerical metrics, and a final part of Latin terms. Their consensus was that there was still no definitive answer for my troubling condition.

Every fresh face required telling the story of the run-up to being in the hospital, so Peggy dutifully recounted the tale as best she could. She started with my morning swim, including the jellyfish sting I'd woefully forgotten to mention until after I had CPR, all the way up to the present moment.

Dr. Ling perked up when she heard a sting, possibly by a jellyfish. She said she'd do some checking and get back to Peggy on that.

Heart of the Journey

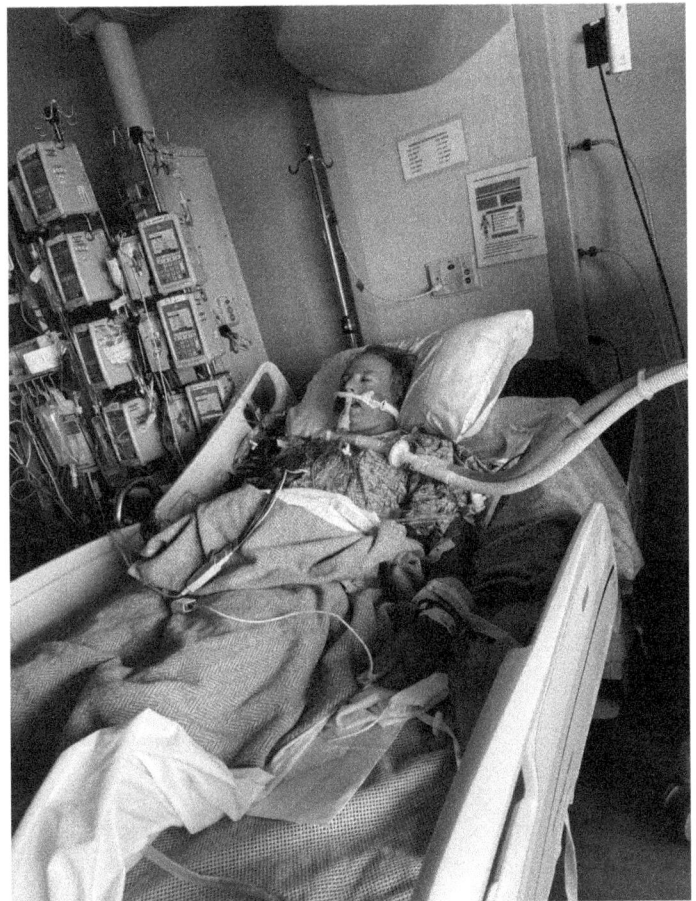

Not at my best

20

A Curious Case

*It's not what happens to you,
but what you do with what happens to you.*

—Anonymous

Saturday, Midday, April 27

By lunchtime on Saturday, the news of whatever was wrong with me had breached, and the family group widened to include friends near and far. Peggy spent most of the day fielding calls and text messages about my condition. Most people in such a situation probably would have cut and pasted the contents of texts that stated general information. But Peggy, being who she is, gave everyone her personal attention. Had I known about the well wishes, I would have been equal parts flattered and embarrassed that everyone was fussing over me so much. But it would be days before I knew what planet I was on.

One downside of being hooked up to ECMO is that there's limited time without life-threatening consequences—but the upside is, your body finally gets the rest it needs. To achieve this, the doctors kept me on propofol, keeping me knocked out while I was hooked into the ECMO and intubated.

With me in la-la land, Peggy focused on fielding calls and chatting with any of the medical team that showed up. One of her rocks was a nurse named Sofia, who started her day shift after I was deposited back in the ICU. One must be an exceptional spirit to work in an ICU. Every day, an ICU nurse can encounter patients who may be experiencing the worst day of their lives. People react differently in these situations—some with anger, others in a state of shock—but an ICU nurse must be prepared for anything.

Unfortunately, not all medical staff have the same calming presence. Many doctors, for instance, aren't inclined to channel their inner Dr. Gregory House, MD, to solve medical mysteries. Most of the time, doctors can interpret test metrics and symptoms to diagnose and treat illnesses. When doctors can't use the surety of data, it's frustrating. This isn't like being unable to figure out what's wrong with a dishwasher—except that the inability to diagnose means someone can lose their life. I cannot fathom how frustrating that would be.

In my case, that frustration spilled over into an early heated debate among the medical team as Dr. Ling, the hospital's infectious disease specialist, engaged in a spirited conversation with Dr. Daniels about my case. The debate wasn't anything like a knock-down, drag-out fight—it was two experienced professionals stating their positions on something neither could prove with absolute certainty. And Peggy was seated ringside for the event.

Dr. Ling thought I had a skin and soft tissue infection brought on by something picked up in the waters from my swim, but she wouldn't commit to speculation beyond that. She thought it would have been missed in the tissue culture, due to its sensitivity to the antibiotics I had been administered earlier.

Meanwhile, Dr. Daniels was convinced that my heart failure had been triggered by a rare envenomation event from a box jellyfish, a condition known as Irukandji syndrome, more specifically. This syndrome is caused by stings from certain small box jellyfish found in tropical Indo-Pacific waters and now seen in places like Hawaii. Symptoms can include delayed onset of severe pain, nausea, vomiting, and, in some cases, life-threatening complications.

Ordinarily, a box jellyfish sting is excruciating—you'd know instantly. But in my case, the sting felt more like a sudden shock. It was definitely noticeable and unlike any jellyfish encounter I'd had before, but it hadn't registered as severe at the time.

Regardless of the cause of my symptoms, the compounded problem was the underlying sepsis I had contracted. Venom and bacteria tend to leave necrotic tissue in their wake. By the time a box jellyfish's venom starts to do visible damage (assuming the unfortunate recipient of the sting hasn't already died), it's already had time to worm its way through the body, releasing little toxin bombs and creating necrotic tissue.

With each passing minute, my body could've been healing itself or sinking deeper into decay. There was one certainty: I couldn't stay on the ECMO forever. Most patients were off the machine within three or four days, at the most. My lactic acid and triglyceride levels were increasing, as were the massive amounts of fluid I was retaining. These were all byproducts of the medications I was on and the side effects of the ECMO.

The doctors needed to figure out what to do with me, and fast.

Saturday Evening, April 27

The staff wasn't going to let Peggy stay in the ICU with me overnight but said she could return during visiting hours. Before she left, she kissed me sweetly on the forehead and whispered, "No drama."

Time would tell.

21

Vail Beginnings

The grass is greener where you water it.
—Anonymous

No one in our circle of friends or family was shocked when Peggy and I got engaged. In fact, they seemed more surprised that we had left the Bay Area, apparently on a one-way ticket. I believe there were even family bets out for when we would decide we'd had enough and would return. I am a fifth-generation San Franciscan, which alone caused confusion as to why I might be thinking about "escaping." Our family and friends were happy for us and supportive, but when we told anyone, it felt like a foregone conclusion that we would eventually get married. I guess that's what happens when you just fit with someone. Everyone else in the world sees how comfortable you are with your partner. In their eyes, you've already formed a partnership, whether you have a certificate, ring, or simple promise to be together.

That's a quaint thought, but 1995 was a busy year for us. We were bound and determined to have our wedding before the end of the year. Just as we settled into our home in Crested Butte, I was being pulled back to California. Gavin Newsom and Billy Getty had another PlumpJack project waiting. They had purchased the Squaw Valley Inn, built in 1960, for the Olympic games that occurred there that year, with the intention of giving it a major renovation and transforming it into a charming mountain retreat with big city hospitality. PlumpJack would become an anchor for countless travelers, skiers, and adventurers, as transformative as any mountain trail.

Returning to California felt like a bit of a detour, but I was used to going where the work took me, and I tried to make the most of it. After all, this was by far the largest and most prominent job I'd had to date. It required me to hire a team of carpenters, craftsmen, and subcontractors to diligently revamp fifty-five guest rooms and suites, along with all the common areas, restaurant, bar, reception, and outside dining areas. It involved working with the Gettys' personal interior design firm, Levitt Weaver, all while trying to keep the budget intact for the discerning, yet young, ownership group.

At the same time, Peggy and I were planning a wedding to occur mid-project. The big day was eventually set for June 3, 1995, outside Vail, Colorado, at a mountaintop resort called Cordillera. That choice felt like the most natural thing in the world to us. Vail was where we could start our story together, in a place that truly represented who we were. Colorado was our middle ground. She was a transplant from Chicago; I, of course, had my roots firmly planted in San Francisco.

We didn't want our wedding to be anything massive or ostentatious. That wasn't us—although, we did have parties in both places to celebrate with those who couldn't make it to Colorado, giving Peggy two more chances to show off a dress you usually only wore once. We tried to keep the main event simple, so we could focus on the step we were taking. The guest list wasn't going to be extensive, either. We'd invite only our closest friends and family.

We chose a destination far enough from both of our worlds, hoping it would filter out casual attendees and leave only those who would truly remain part of our lives as we grew beyond our respective circles.

When the planning was done, all we had to do was wait for the day. That wasn't difficult, as both of us had packed schedules. We went through our day-to-day without much thought about the wedding, or at least I didn't. There were occasional moments when I wondered if anything would change in our relationship once we said, "I do." Relationships can shift simply because of a piece of paper—but mostly for the better, I was convinced. We had a few good arguments while dating that allowed us the chance to show we could work through things and evolve. After that,

I could see no other stumbling blocks in our way. We continued to work when we had to and enjoyed travel and adventures when time allowed. How could I not want that for the rest of my life?

The thoughts of togetherness and adventure were only reinforced when we got to our wedding destination. I still remember standing on that mountaintop, thinking how beautiful it was. The Lodge at Cordillera is perched 8,200 feet above sea level, surrounded by 14,000-foot peaks and the quiet strength of the mountain range. All the scenery was a not-so-subtle nod to stability and permanence—qualities we both admired and wanted to build our lives around.

The morning of the wedding was full of contradictions and had a forecast of rain. On the one hand, I was excited and ready to begin this new chapter with Peggy, but there was also an unexpected sadness and a strange ache. We had been together almost every day since we officially started dating, yet tradition said we shouldn't see each other before the ceremony, except for some photos to be taken beforehand.

Keeping with established wedding-day practice, Peggy had gone off with her friends, doing whatever women do when they get together to prepare for a wedding, which in her case was hiking. I was with buddies, trying to pass the time with a round of golf. I played because I wanted to spend time with my friends, but something was off. While I truly enjoyed their company, what I really wanted was to be near Peggy and the dogs, exploring these gorgeous mountains.

When we were done hacking our way through the links, my buddies shuttled me back to the resort to get ready. I didn't feel nervous until I cut myself shaving. It was just a little nick around my chin, but it felt like a minor catastrophe. A wedding day shouldn't have any cuts or imperfections—right? But there I was, fumbling through the preparations, with my best friends trying to keep me steady.

With the help of my pals, I made it to the ceremony, but so did the rain clouds. I was worried the weather would put a literal damper on our big day, but that all changed when I saw Peggy and her big smile. Shortly after saying our "I dos," a friend from my childhood, Renee, began singing Bette Midler's "From a Distance" and playing guitar. When Renee sang the line

"God is watching us from a distance," a distant clap of thunder rolled as the rain clouds neared—we're not religious, but it was noted.

Then I felt something wet on my cheek. It wasn't raining yet—was it? For a moment, I wondered if it was a shaving nick starting to bleed. How would it look in the wedding pictures if I had a weeping sore on my face? I casually touched my face and then looked down at my fingertips. My digits were wet, all right, but the fluid was clear—and warm. I wasn't bleeding, I was crying. That wasn't something I did often—I didn't tear up in private, let alone in public. Yet there I was, in full view of the crowd, revealing early signs of what some might call a high EQ, or emotional quotient. The rain eventually came and the best man was caught on film looking up and catching a few drops in his mouth, all while I was thinking, *What did I do to deserve having this woman want to spend the rest of her life with me?*

Inside the wedding band I had just placed on Peggy's finger, it read: *John . . .* And inside my band, the inscription read: *. . . I do too.* The engraving was reaching back to a time when Peggy and I were dating, and the word *love* didn't yet come as easy for me as it did for her. Lying in bed one rainy weekend morning as Peggy had started to say "those words," I spoke over her and just gave her the assurance, "I do too." It came off cute at the time and seemed to pacify the moment with understanding and some laughter.

The wedding ceremony ended, and I'm almost positive Peggy was clear-eyed during the whole thing. That was fine with me. I would have hated for her to smudge what little makeup she wore while the photographer snapped pictures.

During the reception, Peggy's stepfather, Chuck Usiskin, gave a fantastic toast. He talked about how incredible it was that we were beginning our life together on a mountaintop and how fitting it felt. And it did—it was like we were already starting higher, aiming higher. I don't know if I fully appreciated it then, but that day's significance has only deepened over the years.

Looking back, I realize that although my friends were happy for me, they hadn't had the chance to know Peggy like I did. She wasn't from their San Francisco-centric world. She was a little quieter than most of my friends, and they hadn't often been around her. I think in my friends' eyes,

Heart of the Journey

our relationship still felt like a bit of a mystery. There wasn't that immediate connection or social comfort that everyone just understood. But to me, that didn't matter. I knew what I'd found in her, and I was confident enough in our bond that I didn't feel the need to justify it.

Before Peggy, my life in San Francisco had followed this perfectly scripted, insular path. I was a part of that city's social fabric, deeply embedded in that world. I'd even taken part in the cotillion circuit three times as an escort—dressed in white tie and tails and paired with a debutante for her ceremonial introduction to society. Looking back, that life seemed like a strange paradox now—I'd been so tied up in that predictable routine, feeling like I knew everyone in town and every hidden alley, busy street, and corner of the city like the back of my hand.

Peggy wasn't drawn to the endless circuit of social events or the carefully curated connections that had defined much of my past. In fact, she didn't conform to what was expected unless she wanted to—she's like her father that way. I was already feeling the pull away from the city scene when I met her, but social circles have a gravity of their own that makes them hard to escape.

I could still be living the life of a bachelor today or could've married into "the scene," convincing myself I would remain content. But then there was Peggy, offering me something I hadn't realized I wanted—a life that felt grounded, real, and uniquely ours. Together, we made a conscious decision to start our own life somewhere else, removed from predictability. We were forced to find friendships and experiences that had meaning to *us*, not inherited expectations or prescribed paths. We wanted the outdoors and a simpler life. Ironically, I believe the success we've built has far outpaced what we might have achieved had we stayed in San Francisco.

Stepping away from known quantities is always risky, but conscious reinvention is also a declaration. Peggy and I were going to live life on our terms. We didn't have the same safety nets or comforts waiting for us in Utah, Colorado, or Idaho. We only had each other, and maybe that's why we're still together today. We're blessed, but not by triumphs or by comparing ourselves to others. We have always measured our success by the life we've built together—and continue to build.

John Baker

A wedding at Cordillera was only the beginning. It was a ceremonial step onto a mountaintop, yes, but also a promise to keep climbing together, even through stormy weather, which did come. Looking back now, I wouldn't change a thing. Colorado was where our life started, and today, it's a reminder of everything we hoped for and everything we've become.

22

Putting Down Roots

Shoot for the moon.
Even if you miss, you'll land among the stars.
—Norman Vincent Peale

While Peggy and I kept the tradition of the groom and bride not seeing each other the morning before the wedding, we ducked the practice of a honeymoon. But skipping a traditional honeymoon didn't feel like a sacrifice to either of us—the decision to wait was a conscious step toward the future we wanted, which was for the rest of our lives together to become an extended honeymoon.

Plus, I was in the thick of one of the most significant projects of my career, and I cannot underscore how big a door opener the PlumpJack project was for me. There was no question about it—this was not a project I could just step away from longer than the wedding itself. This was a leap from my beginnings as a carpenter to general contracting a multi-million-dollar hotel renovation. From remodeling a kitchen for Peggy, here I was, suddenly steering a project of this size and caliber.

Peggy understood. She knew what this opportunity meant for us. Thankfully, the PlumpJack project managed without me for the short time we were gone. Good planning and strict deadlines kept the crews busy in my absence. Later that year, I do recall pausing the project briefly during the afternoon of October 3, 1995, so everyone on the job could watch the final verdict of the OJ Simpson murder trial. It was a big deal back then when the glove just didn't fit! ("If the glove doesn't fit, you must acquit!") I have so many lasting memories of keeping the crews and hotel project moving forward while enjoying moments of our life together in the mountains. After all, it was the journey—not the destination—that truly mattered.

Having connections with Gavin Newsom and Billy Getty was almost worth working for free. The names of the two partners will resonate with anyone who knows the world of California politics and society. Gavin was on his own trajectory back then, and I wouldn't have been surprised to see him in the White House one day. Billy was part of the Getty Oil legacy that had literally fueled America's progress for the last century. No matter how high in politics Gavin rose or what business ventures Billy would go on to back, they were two rare people who trusted me early on.

The faith and trust Gavin and Billy put in me was nothing compared to how much Peggy believed in me. Even when things didn't look as secure as we might have hoped, her resolve never wavered. Her father, like many parents, was a firm believer that a husband (especially his daughter's husband) should offer stability and consistent paychecks. My parents also preferred that same security for me. A regular paying job and something dependable—that's what made sense to our parents.

Peggy saw things a little differently, or at least, she saw the potential I was reaching for. She never gave me grief about taking risks or making unconventional moves. I'll always be grateful to her for that. In those early years, when money was tighter, I had the luxury that she was financially independent in her own right. She never put pressure on me to produce; she never panicked about me putting food on the table. I never leaned on her financially, but knowing she didn't rely on me alone gave me room to grow and take on a little added business risk at times.

I think Peggy's belief in me might have been different had I not constantly been hustling for what came next. I'm a little ashamed to say this, but I saw an opportunity while at Cordillera the day after our wedding. While we were at lunch, I overheard whispers that the company that owned Cordillera was planning further housing development—possibly even another golf course in the area.

When the timing was right, I was able to ask one of the staff, "Who do I need to talk to about this development?" He pointed me in the direction of their construction offices right across the street. It was one of those mountaintop moments when things seemed to align, and fate smiled at me. I walked right over to the offices, climbed a few steps, and found the person in charge of construction management. After a brief introduction and a casual name drop of Gavin, Billy, and the PlumpJack Inn project, the man in charge knew I was legit.

The construction manager started laying out their plans and sharing the vision for this new ground-up project. They were about six months from starting, which would time out perfectly with the projections for finishing the PlumpJack Inn project. It wasn't the timing or even Cordillera's near-mystical setting that sold me on the project—it was the man I spoke with who ran the development business there. I was so impressed with the architecture and quality of the project that I listened to every word he said. By the end of his pitch, I was convinced—this was the next business move I needed. It was a big project, exactly the kind of opportunity I'd been eager to pursue. And best of all, it meant we'd be heading back to Colorado. I knew I had to plant that seed and make sure they saw me as the right person for the job.

I probably didn't talk with Peggy about that interaction on our wedding weekend, but she knew about it in depth long before the PlumpJack project ended, and we moved from Lake Tahoe back to Crested Butte. That wouldn't be the only time we moved or found temporary accommodations. We moved around a lot to go where the projects led me. Sometimes, with gaps between projects, we felt more settled socially, but job insecurity always crept in for me. That kind of lifestyle takes its toll, even if you're making money along the way.

But once the PlumpJack hotel project was wrapped up in January of 1996, we knew we wanted to go back to the Rocky Mountains, regardless of whether the Cordillera project came to fruition. Crested Butte was still calling, and as soon as we could, we found our way back. The juggling, planning, and logistics didn't bother us. My life in the Colorado mountains had a pull that felt magnetic. It was where we thought we wanted to live our life together.

After a short time in Crested Butte, the networking seeds I'd planted on my wedding weekend sprouted. I secured the contract to build a clubhouse for Cordillera's Valley Club—notably, the course was designed by my favorite modern day golf course architect, Tom Fazio. The project was another milestone and another leap. So later that year, we packed up once again, heading for Edwards, Colorado. Our family was growing—now with three big dogs, including Bradley the Newfoundland. We bought a townhome where we hoped to finally stay put for a year or two.

In some ways, these moves felt like the honeymoon we'd missed. Every time we relocated for a new project, it was a fresh start—new locations and the thrill of taking on larger projects. For each transition, we leaned on our faith and confidence in one another and ourselves. Peggy, for her part, was always willing to go along with these moves. She understood my drive and my need to test the limits, and she embraced it with a kind of steady trust.

Peggy wasn't just along for the ride. She saw a purpose in all those moves, all those temporary homes. We were building something more than a business; we were building a future together. We were buying real estate where we could, making improvements, and planting acorns that we knew would eventually show returns. I was probably more driven by that vision than I realized at the time. We didn't have to own property in Edwards, but it was part of the bigger plan. We were building equity in our lives and our future, treating each house or project as part of a broader vision.

Over time, I began to see the beauty of passive income. I once heard an old-school landlord refer to passive income as "mailbox money." That's rent or an investment coming in with no more effort than going out to the mailbox and getting a check. Not all real estate has a mailbox money component. Some deals, like the spec house I built later on, are a one-and-done proposition. You put the time and effort in for the hopes of one big payday.

Peggy and I have always been hands-on and focused with our investments, making certain they offer strong returns. For every good income year we had, we reinvested. We didn't want to just "get by." We wanted our future to flourish on its own terms. And now, all these years later, we are at a point where the interest on our investments is more than we need. The plan worked even better than I could've hoped. The roots we planted in those early years took hold, blossoming into a life of security and stability we can appreciate together.

Getting back to our missed honeymoon, we did plan something later—a sailing trip through Greece and Turkey that I was going to somehow captain myself. However, again, the trip never materialized, because Peggy's stepfather Chuck fell ill and suddenly needed a liver and kidney transplant.

We dropped everything to be there for Chuck, and for Peggy's mother, Dorothy, because being there for them mattered. In the grand scheme of things, the honeymoon felt small in comparison. Life had a way of throwing curveballs, but it also reminded you where your priorities should lie.

23

Lessons in Life Balance

Easy choices, hard life. Hard choices, easy life.
—Anonymous

One of the more significant turning points of my career came not in the chaos of the construction site or the calculated calm of a real estate deal, but in the shimmering luxury of Monte Carlo. It began midway through the Cordillera project in the winter of 1996.

With the title of general contractor, I was perpetually accountable to someone else. It was an existence I'd long questioned. From the moment I first strapped on a tool belt, I had dreamed of being my own boss. I wanted to call the shots, and I wasn't the type of person who thought owning my own business would be rosy and pain-free. By the time I was in high school and Griff Towle and I went rogue, staining houses in Lake Tahoe, I was ready to take responsibility for the risks and rewards of being captain of my own ship.

Yet, the reality of contracting often felt like the antithesis of that dream. Every project meant answering someone else's vision, deadlines, and demands. The pressure to deliver was at times unrelenting, and sometimes the stakes were too high when balancing the rewards. When you're pushing construction crews who are living hand to mouth for near unreasonable results, there's a higher price to pay. But that butcher's bill wouldn't come until after Monte Carlo in the fall of 1996.

Heart of the Journey

When Peggy told me about her father's sixtieth birthday celebration in Monte Carlo, my primitive brain thought she was going alone. *John's in work mode. John has no time for Monte Carlo.* This was what my single-track mind thought in response to her announcing the event. However, I could tell that it was important to her. Once I stepped out of my work shoes, I realized it mattered to me, too. Jim was a savvy businessman who worked hard for everything he had. As part of the family, I should be there to share in the fruits of his labors and to celebrate this milestone in his life.

Plus, several days of opulence awaited us. I never want to admit that I need a break from work, but once we sat in our flight's business-class seats surrounded by Peggy's family, I felt how tired I'd been. As the flight progressed, my mind slowly drifted away from work. I'd planned everything I could for my absence. I had to trust that those I put in charge would execute their duties the same as if I were standing nearby. If not, I'd clean up any messes when I got back. I could do nothing about it, so I might as well enjoy the ride.

Monte Carlo was a shimmering jewel perched above the Mediterranean. Every turn exuded opulence, from Casino de Monte-Carlo to the yachts gleaming in the harbor. The city was a playground for those who had mastered life's high stakes. It had an air of untouchable exclusivity designed for only the boldest and richest of dreamers. We had hotel accommodations that redefined any concept I had of luxury. We dined in gilded halls, drank wine older than I was, and strolled streets that whispered of old money and ambition fulfilled. It was intoxicating—and unsettling.

When the trip was over, I was glad I'd taken the mental respite, but coming home to Vail was like being wrenched from a dream. One day, I was clinking glasses with the privileged; the next, I was back on the jobsite in jeans encrusted with drywall dust, working alongside people whose lives had been shaped more by hands-on experience than formal education. There was nothing wrong with being a tradesperson—it was a skilled and often noble profession. But I couldn't help wondering why I seemed to have a broader vision than many of those I employed. Was it the advantages I'd been given, the lessons my parents instilled in me, or was it just something innate?

I remember staring at my boots one morning with the echoes of Monte Carlo still fresh in my mind and thinking, *This is unsustainable.* The stark divide between those two worlds—the difference between the affluence of those surroundings and the grinding reality of my own—was too great. The realization hit me like a moment of clarity: I didn't want to just watch others experience financial success and the freedoms that came with it. I wanted to earn it, possess it, and live it fully. But turning points don't happen without elements of chaos attached—and that bedlam would come two days later.

I'll never forget the day it happened. It was a beautiful clear morning, and the crew was busy framing the interiors of the new golf clubhouse while I was reviewing plans in the trailer. Everything seemed to be going smoothly until I heard a scream. At first, I thought someone had just hit their finger with a hammer or was screaming out in sheer frustration. I immediately ran into the building to assess the situation. One of the framers had been using a skill saw to cut a piece of wood when the saw suddenly caught the wood and jerked it violently. His hand was pulled forward into the spinning blade before he had time to react. Three of his fingers were severed completely, and blood was splattered across him and the nearby walls.

It wasn't like those movie scenes where kidnappers cut off someone's finger to send it as a message. Those scenes are filled with shots of the kidnappers' near-disgust at having to go to those lengths. That wasn't the case here. The crew was capriciously calm. Moreover, I wasn't freaking out, either. This crisis was just like any other—assess, respond, and report. Then, I realized that everyone else on the construction site was trauma-bonded, because we'd seen our share of accidents.

Anyone who's been on a construction site for long knows close calls are just part of the job. Thinking back, there had been more than I cared to count—ladders that had slipped out from under me, saws that came terrifyingly close to slicing off my fingers, objects ejected from table saws nearly striking my eye. Each near-miss had been just plain luck, but I congratulated myself for being either cunning or fortunate enough to live another day. Not until the day I saw fingers lying on the floor did I think,

Damn, doing this is pretty precarious, and my ticket is going to get punched eventually. I realized I didn't need to be the kind of boss who was up on the ladder anymore. I could be the guy who hired the company, who employed the guy on that ladder. After all, Peggy and I were just months away from having our first child, so we didn't need any unnecessary risks—I had more than just myself to think about now.

For years, I'd built my reputation as a general contractor by being on-site and in the mix, always the first to show up and the last to leave. But staring at the bloodied scene, I knew this was no longer just about managing jobs or proving my worth. There was a tension I hadn't expected between who I was professionally and who I needed to become. I had to make peace with stepping away—not because I didn't care, but because I cared too much to keep going the same way. It was a fundamental shift in mindset from being indispensable on the jobsite to being irreplaceable in a different sense: setting a vision, creating opportunities, and being truly in charge.

That day marked the pivot point. My role evolved from contractor to conductor, from hands-on builder to strategic developer. I wasn't just laying foundations for others anymore; I was now investing in futures, starting with my own.

This shift in late 1997 wasn't just because of Monte Carlo and the allure of financial independence. The less time I spent on single jobsites, the more time I could spend making deals and setting up more projects. I was tired of asking permission to take time off, of feeling guilty for enjoying a life I hadn't yet built for myself. Something had to give, and it was clear I would have to step away from the iron grip of general contracting.

Freedom comes with its challenges. As I tried to find my way over the next several years, the stress didn't vanish—it morphed. Gone was the steady income of completing one project at a time and then questioning what was next. In its place came irregular windfalls and the constant quest to build a steady portfolio of commercial properties. But I'd take that bit of uncertainty over the soul-crushing grind of contracting any day.

Looking back, Monte Carlo and all it represented wasn't just a trip or a turning point in my career. It was a defining moment that forced me to confront the gap between the life I was living and the life I wanted. It gave me the push to say, "Enough!" I wanted to leave hands-on management behind, step into the real estate world, and start building a legacy. It wasn't an overnight transformation, but the start of something bigger—a life on my terms.

And for that, I'll always be thankful.

24

Terry

Age is just a number.
—Anonymous

When it comes to life on my own terms, I had big shoes to fill. While many of my friends, and even Peggy, experienced the death of their elderly, eighty-something-year-old parents, my grandmother on my mother's side not only lived to over 106 but thrived with dignity. I gladly made the time to call her regularly, and whenever I was in San Francisco, visiting her was a priority. Her name was Theresa Breyer, but she went by Terry.

She was an inspiration to me. Her mind remained sharp, and she stayed engaged with the world through current events and reading the paper. It became part of her identity. She often reminded us of her age, playfully saying she had kept it a secret from everyone in her building. There's a saying, "Age is just a number," but Terry was rewriting the rules—she was determined to get the best of life. She not only inspired me to focus on meaningful conversations with others but also to stay healthy.

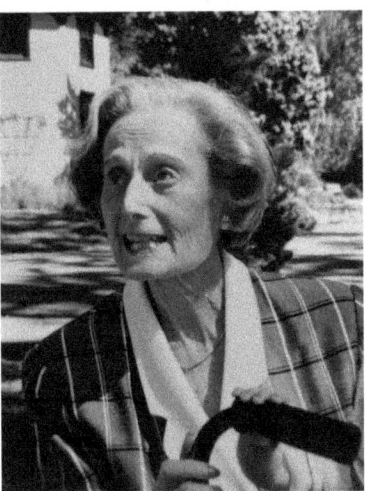

My grandmother, Terry, showing some glamour

"Grandma, I just finished my fifth New York Marathon and had my personal best time!"

Her silence left me puzzled, but finally a response came.

"Stop running."

More puzzled now, I politely inquired for more information.

"If you plan to walk in your later years, you should stop running."

She had a point. There was really nothing more that needed to be said. In November 2019, I ran my fifth and final marathon. Swimming would be the next sport for my cardio health.

She always started her day by dressing properly. Never would you find her in a bathrobe. She took pride in her appearance and dignity, wearing her favorite St. John outfits, always in practical colors with modest jewelry or a cashmere outfit with a matching cardigan.

My last visit with her was in March 2022.

"Grandma, you look tired," I said.

"I didn't sleep well last night."

"What happened?" I asked, expecting to hear about an ache or a side effect from medication.

"I just didn't want to miss anything!" she said with a slight smile.

Even at 106 years old, Terry was clear: She wanted to stay engaged with life. One of the more important things we can do for the elderly is to listen. Too often, we see them through stereotypes instead of as individuals with unique experiences.

Years earlier, for her 100th birthday, we celebrated in the back room at Harris' Restaurant, a steakhouse in San Francisco, with her three children and several of us grandchildren. I was honored to sit beside her. We talked about how difficult it was for her to give up her seventh-floor apartment and move into assisted living on the lower level. Like most things, she wanted it to happen on her terms and needed time to adjust. I deeply understood her need for independence—it was something that we shared. I've always valued the ability to make my own decisions and set my own course. While I can go with the flow when there's someone trustworthy at the helm, more often than not, I've felt the need to be that person myself.

Terry was independent and strong-willed, rare qualities for a woman born in the early 1900s. She lost her husband, my grandfather, Stanley Breyer, in 1975, when she was only fifty-eight. She remarried in 1979 but outlived her second husband as well. Surviving on her own for decades made her fiercely independent, a trait some family members struggled to understand. But I admired it.

She prioritized social connections, always making plans for meals or bridge games. Since she outlived most of her contemporaries, it wasn't unusual for her dinner companions to be younger couples in their seventies. She was more informed about local sports than I was, providing updates on the Forty-Niners or Warriors teams. Whether she did it because she thought I followed sports or because she truly cared, I was never sure—but she was always prepared with conversation starters, a skill I came to appreciate and practice myself.

Terry had an unspoken rule: No talk of politics or health issues. "We all have aches and pains," she said, "so why sit around and hear the same old complaints?" She saw such topics as unworthy of quality conversation. Even as I moved into my fifties and sixties, I took that to heart and tried not to whine about a sore back from golfing or leg cramps from running. She taught me to embrace discomfort as part of life and to engage with people in more meaningful ways.

A friend once asked me, "What's her secret?"

"She goes through life in moderation," I replied. "She also avoids politics and health complaints. She prefers to talk about family and friendships."

He nodded in understanding.

"And good genes don't hurt," I added.

Terry outlived two husbands and all of her friends, living a full and meaningful life until she passed in 2022. We should all hope to have such a clear mind as hers as we age.

Reflecting on my relationships, I've always found it easier to connect with the women in my life. Perhaps it's because they tend to be more thoughtful, or maybe because I prefer listening to talking. Whatever the reason, this affinity shaped my deep relationships with both of my grandmothers.

While my grandfathers were engaging in their own right, my grandmothers created space for deeper conversations. Virginia and Terry each left a unique imprint on my life, but both shared the rare gift of making me feel heard. With them, I could open up in ways I couldn't with others. As a listener by nature, I felt comforted by their thoughtful, attentive communication, which shaped my own communication style. They taught me the value of genuine connection, of making space for others to share their thoughts and feelings. These lessons have served me well, from raising my children to building relationships in business.

My grandmothers showed me that, sometimes, the most meaningful connections come not from what we say, but from how we listen. Their influence lives on in the way I approach relationships today, always remembering that the greatest gift we can give someone is our time and understanding.

25

The Waiting Game

*After being a target, are you defeated,
scared, and branded, or empowered?*

—Martin Short

10:00 a.m., Sunday, April 28

As I lay in a hospital bed in San Francisco—ironically just a few blocks from where Terry had spent the last twenty years of her life—I remained under medically induced sedation. With little to do on Saturday or Sunday, Peggy spent most of her time wrangling the many visitors who had come to see me, starting with family. Wilson and Blair got in late Saturday night and came to see me first thing in the morning, anxiously waiting in the hospital lobby until visiting hours started. It's always unsettling to visit someone in the hospital, but this visit came with added unease: The outcome was far from certain.

When they walked in, they recognized me as their father, but it felt like looking at a stranger lying there on the hospital bed. They were used to my excitement at seeing them, of me fulfilling the role of parent with stoicism, certainty, and stability. Peggy had shown them a picture before entering the room, but nothing could prepare them for actually being there, the reality hitting them like a wave. Their automatic response was to be overcome with tears as they slowly eased into the room.

Holding my hand, Blair didn't know what to say, while Wilson repeated, "You've got this, Dad—keep fighting, Dad." He was committed to taking on the role usually reserved for a parent—one of strength and support.

My brother Chris and my parents made it by lunchtime on Sunday. Peggy's stepsister, Deidre, was also in the mix, along with shorter visitations from a few close San Francisco friends. I'm glad they were all there to form a support network for Peggy.

There's nothing worse than waiting. That Sunday, my family and friends could do nothing but watch over me during my propofol-induced slumber. In TV shows and movies, they always focus on the beeps the machinery makes, implying that regular noise adds to the stress of the situation. In my case, the beeping was fine—it let everyone know that at least the machinery keeping me alive was functioning correctly.

The room had soft sage walls and dim lighting, aimed at bringing comfort to those watching a loved one go through an experience they might not survive. There was no clear delineation between the room and the outside hallways, and this detail was particularly unnerving to my family. It suggested that those in these rooms were so unstable that the turning of a doorknob could be the difference between life and death.

The far side of the room is where my family kept vigil; they sat in a row of chairs, like an audience waiting for my next act. Next to them was a small window that provided the sparse amount of sunlight that lit the room.

I was flanked by various machines. To my right was the machine connected to my intubation, exhaling rhythmic breath sounds and beeps. To my left was a wall of tubes that provided me with the unique antibiotic cocktail designed to attack anything that was possibly causing my mysterious illness.

Sunday Afternoon, April 28

A curious thing was happening during this time. Even with IV medications being administered, the "curtain of comfort" would gradually lift as the anesthetic began to fade, if only briefly, before settling back in again. It was during this hazy time that I can recall the comforting voice of my mother while she held my hand, recounting pleasant memories of recent time we'd spent together in New York's Central Park—or the comforting voice of a high school friend named Bronwyn, wishing me strength to recover. It was these calm voices that resonated, offering me peace.

The good news at that stage was that my readings were more stable. They had pumped me with so much fluid and drugs that I was retaining twenty-seven pounds of them. My fingers were swollen up like Vienna sausages that had been left outside on a hot summer day. Luckily, Peggy had the foresight to remove my wedding ring before it was too late. She wore it on a chain around her neck for a while, then on her finger below her wedding ring band.

The swelling couldn't go on forever. The more fluid I retained, the harder it would be for my heart and lungs to function. I would need to be taken off the ECMO and extubated soon, but when and how that would happen was yet to be determined; I think the medical staff was waiting for Monday morning to roll around. As wonderfully dedicated as those who work in hospitals are, weekends are usually when the B team shines. All the medical heavy hitters and decision-makers would look at my case on Monday morning.

Monday Morning, April 29

The decision was carefully made to begin weaning me off the propofol due to my elevated triglyceride levels. However, it wasn't until several long hours later, at exactly 1:32 p.m., that the doctors actually started the process. Waking me up was supposed to be the prelude to removing the ECMO and ventilator that had become the silent overseers of my survival. Much to my dismay, what we thought would take mere hours stretched into an agonizing thirty-hour delay.

Without a doubt, lying in that bed—reawakened and now conscious, yet connected to the lifesaving machines—was the most challenging time of my life. Imagine drifting into one of those deep Sunday afternoon naps, the kind that leaves you groggy and disoriented when you wake, unsure of what day or time it is. Now, take that feeling and multiply it, because when

I woke up, I hadn't just lost track of time—I had lost control of my body. My memory was picture-perfect until the moment I got on the plane in Hawaii. But when I was lucid enough to understand I'd actually lost three days of my life, it shook me. If emotions are internal signals helping us evaluate situations, my signals were flashing red due to an apparent power failure. The intersection was a confusing mix of thinking about what I should do next versus just yielding to the oncoming situation at hand.

Looking around, I could clearly see my family gathered around my bed while I was restrained, intubated, and tethered to the ECMO machine—an overwhelming situation that was nearly too much for me to bear. As I lay there helpless, the sheer weight of my emotions was suffocating. If emotions are at the heart of communication, then the tears welling up in my eyes must have been broadcasting a powerful signal as they pooled and stung. The salty drops constantly streaking my cheeks were a physical reminder of my helplessness until someone provided the needed tissue. If I could speak, there would've been no words in those moments. All I knew was that the hand that had once held others' now needed to be held.

Throughout all this, my kids remained stoic pillars of strength. They refused to crumble under the heavy weight of what they were witnessing. I was in awe of their courage, even as I grappled with the sight of myself in such a weakened, vulnerable state. I wasn't even a fraction of the strong, active man they had always known. If I were a shadow, at least I could have sat up in bed, but no—I was a helpless mass, stripped of even the most basic freedoms.

I understand why they had my body locked down, but that didn't help much. If I were to have any involuntary body movements, common with patients on propofol, I might pull the ECMO tubes out. I also had the risk of getting confused and pulling out my ventilator tube. I imagined that if those tubes got pulled, it would be a huge problem in a matter of seconds. I wouldn't be able to breathe. I didn't know how long it would take me to suffocate, but I didn't want to find out. I lay there as still as I could, powerless, helpless, but mostly scared. One of my first thoughts coming out of my induced slumber was, *Am I about to die?*

Heart of the Journey

I'm certain this ordeal was far worse for my wife and children, as I remember catching snippets of conversation between the doctors and Peggy. "We'll deal with his foot later," one of them said. They assured her it wasn't a priority, but that offered little comfort, especially since I didn't fully grasp what was happening. To make matters worse, the intubation tube down my throat left me unable to speak.

After I had been awake for several hours, my medical team finally felt comfortable removing my restraints. They must have sensed from my calm demeanor that I could be trusted not to pull out the many uncomfortable, life-supporting tubes. With the restraints removed, I was finally able to communicate to my family on a pad of paper. Written communication became my lifeline.

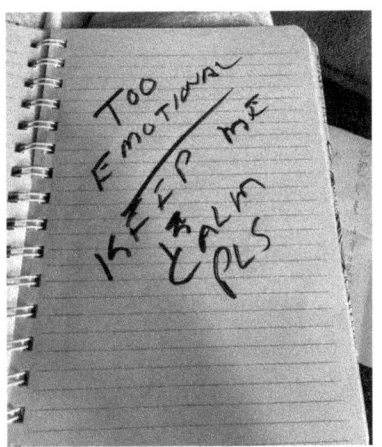

Written messages were my only form of communication during this troubling time

I couldn't talk, but I scribbled cryptic messages to Peggy, Blair, and Wilson. Sometimes, I added pictures to make my thoughts more transparent. My handwriting was shaky and prone to mistakes, and it often resulted in jumbled letters. But Blair had a sixth sense, finishing my sentences as though reading my mind. In those moments, I clung to the fragments of normalcy they brought, even as my reality felt anything but typical.

At first, my questions focused on my mortality: What happened? How did I end up here? Was I going to survive? But while my family lived in the euphoria of my liveliness, I couldn't help but ask about market prices and various business affairs. What had I missed in those few days? It may seem trivial compared with what was at stake, but these questions were part of a long mental process of slowly piecing the puzzle back together.

7:00 p.m., Monday, April 29

Before Peggy and the kids left the hospital for the night, she leaned in close and said again, as she had before, "Stay strong. No drama tonight."

Wilson, ever the cheerleader, added, "You got this."

I latched onto their words, using them as a mantra to get through what became the longest night of my life. With visitation hours over at 7:00 p.m., I was left alone with my thoughts, an analog clock on the wall, and the rhythmic hum of the machines keeping me alive. Knowing there were people on the other side of this fight who were waiting, hoping, and praying for me gave me a reason to keep pushing through the uncertainty—but this was different. This was a silent endurance. I couldn't speak due to the intubation, so I had to rely on my eyes and slight movements to communicate with caregivers. Every nod, every squeeze of a hand, became my language of determination. Just as I'd learned through running, during this longest night of my life, the only way through was to focus on the finish line, not the agony of it all.

I don't wish upon anyone the frustration that plagued me Monday night into Tuesday. I don't want you or anyone else in the world to have an inkling of the mental pain and despair of being alone, tied to a bed. It was bad enough that, a few times, I wondered if it wouldn't be better to die. Every horrible scenario can turn into a fixation for a mind that has nothing to latch onto but discomfort.

I was still trying to remember what had gotten me here, piecing together the mystery of it all as well as replaying the day's events and conversations I'd overheard from my family. I couldn't help but question my life's decisions and the value I'd brought to my family, my business, and the world. Did I create and give back more than I consumed personally or professionally? Did I do a good job passing what I had learned to the next generation? Would I live to do anything about those things if I had fallen short? I stayed awake well into the night, acknowledging the severity of my situation, thankful to be alive, and wondering if life would ever return to the way it was before.

8:00 a.m., Tuesday, April 30

Tuesday morning, before visiting hours, the doctors offered another glimmer of hope: I might be extubated and have the ECMO machine removed soon. But that hope faded again just as quickly as they explained there were established protocols and other patients in critical care on our floor to factor in. My case needed unanimous approval from all the doctors involved before anything could move forward. There wasn't much to do but continue to wait. The ventilator—a painful, invasive tube lodged deep in my throat—was relentless in its torment. It irritated my airway, triggering violent coughing fits that caused the monitors to blare as though signaling my imminent demise. The day stretched ahead like another marathon, one I was not sure I had the strength to finish.

10:00 a.m., Tuesday, April 30

Peggy, Blair, and Wilson returned as soon as visiting hours allowed. Hayden arrived as well, after completing exams. They were ready to advocate for my extubation and the removal of the ECMO. Hours turned into more waiting hours, and doubt began to creep in.

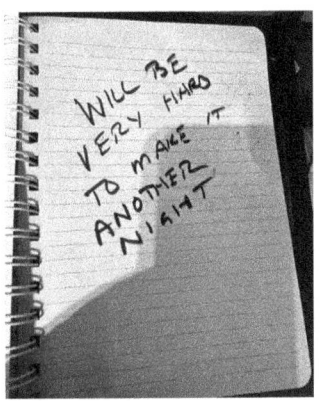

Written message revealing a low point

As I witnessed the team of doctors outside my ICU room, their lips moving but with no words that could be heard, I started to wonder if they were withholding something. Perhaps my condition was worse than they were letting on. I wrote a message in a small notebook that got my point across: "My leg needs drugs, hurts," and "Will be very hard to make it another night."

4:00 p.m., Tuesday, April 30

I doubt my family had any real influence in accelerating the process, but the cardiac team eventually received all the necessary approvals and arrived at my bedside, ready to remove the breathing tubes and ECMO machine. It felt like Navy SEAL Team Six, led by Dr. David Daniels, had assembled around me. I instinctively looked at each one of them, pausing for a moment to let them know with my eyes that I was going to fight alongside them.

Before the team pushed my bed down the hall to the elevator and onto the basement cath lab, an anesthesiologist greeted me with a large dose of ketamine—yes, ketamine. I may have tried a mild psychedelic back in college once, but this was a whole new level. I vividly remember the surreal trip—sliding into a spiraling, Candy Cane Lane-style elevator and arriving in a room filled with magic acts and rock and roll music. There, a team of magicians performed the delicate procedure to remove the ECMO tubes and ventilator. There is no question that the unsung heroes during this time were again Dr. Daniels and his team, who successfully performed this lifesaving surgery.

While I was under, they did another exploratory surgery on my right foot to see if there were any obvious signs of infection eating away at muscle and skin tissue from the inside out. Fortunately, the procedure didn't reveal any new areas of concern; however, we were still no closer to solving the medical mystery behind the extensive damage to my foot.

Tuesday Evening, April 30

I was finally off the ECMO machine, but I still had enormous, open lacerations on my right foot. I accepted this mess would most certainly leave a few battle scars and that I'd likely be unable to walk for some time. That was okay; scars would make a good visual aid for telling the story (if I ever got out of the hospital, that is). The latest ECMO removal and foot surgery meant another three days of being heavily monitored in the ICU, bringing me to Thursday, May 3.

After being unshackled from the ventilator and ECMO machine, I at least felt like I had some control over my body, but it didn't feel like the body I had left behind three days before. Every time I ate or drank anything, it felt like I was swallowing tiny, jagged pebbles. I couldn't move from the bed because of the incisions in my foot and leg. However, I'd take it over the helplessness of being fully tethered to machines, entirely at their mercy. Pain, at least, was something I could feel—something that reminded me I was alive and fighting. It felt too soon to think about what life might look like afterward. But I knew those thoughts would begin to surface in the days ahead.

"Mr. Baker, what is your pain level?" a nurse from the ICU would ask before administering a dose of oxy or fentanyl. Everyone was moving purposefully throughout the unit. Visitors spoke in hushed tones and nearly tiptoed around. I wondered if everyone thought an overly loud voice or turn of phrase would inflict a mortal wound on the patients. In the dim lights, there was no view of the busy city that existed just beyond the walls.

26

Our Early Sun Valley Years

We don't always think alike, but we think together.
—Anonymous

The passing of time is a fantastic stretch. It felt as if one day, I was married in 1995, and the next, we were packing up to move to Sun Valley in November 1997. However, that decision didn't come without many visits and lengthy discussions about which mountain town would be best for us.

We took pride in the fact that we had made our way through many of the western mountain towns. They all had their uniqueness. Telluride was scenic and beautiful, but we felt there was some tension between the haves and the have nots. A mountaintop destination resort with a local town below seemed to create a sense of disparity among the residents. Park City's easy access was a blessing and a curse. Lake Tahoe was just an extension of the Bay Area with its weekend warriors. Same for Vail, but it had a highway running right through the middle, and the hum of a highway is one of my pet peeves. Crested Butte was idyllic in so many ways, but far too remote, and it appeared most people lived there to ski, as they should. Aspen was a civilized mountain town, but the millionaires were moving out, making room for the billionaires to move in. Then, there was Sun Valley. Peggy and I had visited the town several times together and liked what it had to offer.

Sun Valley, nestled in the heart of Idaho's Sawtooth Mountains, radiates a rugged yet polished charm. The destination holds a quiet sophistication, echoing the stories of Hemingway and generations of dreamers seeking solace in its breathtaking solitude. All of these were reasons we were drawn to it and its four distinct seasons—plus, who doesn't like a town with the word Sun in its name? Its snow-draped peaks draw skiers from around the world. That, along with skiing as an amenity, rather than the main event, checked a box for me. High desert, long summers, and a walkable town with everything in reach were real pluses, and Peggy had the vision to realize a good school and well-funded hospital were equally important. We both believed we would find like-minded, healthy individuals with professional careers who shared similar family values there as well.

Idaho's golden summers transformed the valleys into playgrounds for us. In many ways, it was the perfect place for our growing family—a town steeped in outdoor activity yet grounded in a small-town atmosphere. Outside of schooling, our kids would spend their days skiing, hiking, and growing up in an environment as demanding as it was beautiful. We spent the next twenty-five years in Idaho watching our children do just that. Locals have a saying about Sun Valley: "The worst thing about Sun Valley is that it's hard to get to. And the best thing about Sun Valley . . . is that it's hard to get to."

I can imagine the early days, when Sun Valley Ski Resort first opened in 1936—the echoes of laughter in the air as skiers raced down the slopes only to be brought back up the mountain by the first ski lift in the country. This same ski lift now resides on Rudd Mountain, behind our current home. When Peggy and I made the move to this small mountain town, we had no idea what would unfold. But one thing was sure: The outdoor adventure would only be a sideshow, because the biggest adventure of all would be starting a family.

I remember being overwhelmed with joy at the arrival of our firstborn—a daughter I would read stories to and one day learn from. As a father, there are no words to fully express that moment, nor any way to truly prepare for the miracle of life we would both grow to appreciate together.

Blair arrived on February 6, 1998, at 2:44 in the afternoon. The timing couldn't have been more perfect—literally. Peggy, exhausted from a long labor, agreed to have her Pitocin dosage increased, which helped move things along. As it turned out, our obstetrician had a 4:30 p.m. appointment, later revealed to be a haircut, so he was equally motivated in an awkward way to keep things on schedule. In the end, it made for a good story and gave us just a little more time with Blair on this earth, which felt like a gift from the very start.

Notably, while Peggy has several groups of close friends, the one that stands out most is her baby playgroup. It began as a small gathering of young mothers, each celebrating the arrival of their first child. Today, Peggy affectionately refers to Justine, Mary, and Mary Anne as her "Hailey Group," since all but Peggy now live in Hailey, Idaho. They've seen each other weekly since 1998, usually over "coffee." As I write this, those babies, including Blair, are now twenty-seven years old.

The first winter in Sun Valley was everything we hoped for. The idea of raising our children here felt like a dream we could actually hold: snow-capped peaks, endless trails, and a tight-knit community all around us which tied in nicely with the family values that have been important to us.

***

When we first moved to Sun Valley, I volunteered twice a week at Blaine Manor in Hailey, Idaho, a senior care housing facility. It always gave me pleasure to share stories with the elderly or check on their general wellbeing. I was even talked into running their Friday afternoon bingo a few times.

The elderly often get overlooked and may feel like unwanted outsiders in society. Sadly, many participate in their own invisibility by withdrawing into isolation. Volunteering there was my way of both honoring and connecting with wiser souls, and of filling the void of my grandmother Virginia Baker, whom I had recently lost at the age of ninety-two. On one occasion at Blaine Manor, I visited a woman in her nineties, who had just lost her husband after their seventieth wedding anniversary.

"How are you doing?" I asked.

"Well, not everyone can say they were married that long," she said, her voice trailing off. She then looked me in the eye. "Tell me about what's going on with you."

I talked about my business interests, the birth of our first child, and my young marriage.

She nodded, then said, "John, what you get out of marriage is what you put into it."

I looked at her and noticed that though her speech was halting, she had leaned forward.

"The grass is always greener where you water it," she said.

Her comment had the effect of grounding me. I didn't want to move on from what she'd said. I wanted to soak it in. But when I gave her a goodbye and walked out into the hallway, I realized that what I'd witnessed was one of the special aspects of connecting with the elderly. In business, we would consider it an asset. That asset is wisdom, and to be able to tap into that wisdom, one must be patient.

It reminded me of my own grandparents and made me even more grateful for the regular phone calls I had made over the years. Staying connected became even more of a priority once we had relocated to Sun Valley. Despite the time zones or busy days, I made a point to check in with my family members regularly, especially my remaining grandmother Terry, sometimes just to say hi, sometimes to listen. I realized that intentionality is what keeps families close, especially when life pulls everyone in different directions.

***

There are a few things in life that came naturally to me. Fatherhood was not something that I was instantly good at, whereas Peggy was a natural at being a mom. You've seen the videos of some six-year-old kid walking up to a piano and instinctively playing an intricate piece of classical music. Peggy was the same with motherhood. For her, it was almost like flipping a switch—she was a whirlwind of organization and discipline, focused on getting everything just right. She was type A, no question, a woman who could see the future unfolding before anyone else could even finish making a plan. She was confident in her decisions, in how she'd raise Blair, and in doing things the way she felt was right.

Peggy seemed like a child-raising savant, while I was more like her slow-to-learn assistant. The early years of parenthood were nothing like I expected. Then again, what part of life is ever what we expect? When Blair came into our lives, everything shifted. I played the role of the supportive partner—the helper. I was there, but I mostly took a supporting role in parenting. Peggy had it covered. She had a plan, and I had my hands full just trying to keep up. She would famously say, "If the kids aren't kept on a strict daily schedule, then she'd have to pay for their tantrums the next day."

It was around this time, September 1998, that I took on a project for Peggy's brother Charlie Mills and his wife, Kristen. They were midway through an extensive remodel of a large estate home in Lake Forest, Illinois, when they began to lose confidence in their general contractor and his ability to properly complete their home. My commitment to both of them and the project was truly needed. However, it came at the cost of taking me away from Peggy and our newborn, Blair, for six months.

This job required me to wear many hats. First and foremost, I was tasked with firing the general contractor, along with many of his subcontractors, and rehiring new subs that could perform at high standards in short order. Additionally, I was challenged to walk the tightrope of managing my brother and sister-in-law, who were at odds with each other on budget, timing, and quality. It was a leap of faith for them to trust that I could jumpstart this delicate project, along with personally stepping back to play the general contractor role. The project became intense at times. There was even a time I actually fainted and needed to be taken to the hospital for fluids. I must have neglected to hydrate that stressful day and paid the price. Luckily, just a scare.

At times, I felt like more of a marriage counselor than a general contractor, but after all, it's one of the quiet job descriptions of the profession. In reflection, I realized I was, in fact, proficient at orchestrating the many delicate intricacies that go into a successful building project—qualities that I would carry forward into my commercial business but didn't necessarily translate into good parenting or husbandry. However, my absence during this time did show my wife's resilience and support of my career.

Heart of the Journey

Toward the end of the project, I flew home for a long weekend, routing from Chicago O'Hare to Boise, Idaho, for the two-hour drive to Sun Valley. I was exhausted, and as soon as we reached cruising altitude, I drifted into a much-needed sleep.

Several hours later, I was gently stirred awake by a subtle shift in the plane's speed. Nothing alarming at about 30,000 feet, but enough to make me glance out the window on my right to get my bearings. What I saw pulled me into quiet awe—the vast beauty of the Rocky Mountains stretched below, rugged and majestic. I blinked. Were we over Colorado? Wyoming? Already in Idaho?

As I rubbed my eyes, I noticed an idyllic valley coming into view—rolling mountains folding into a modest, green basin and a river winding gracefully through it all. It looked like paradise, exactly as I had imagined it so many times before: the place I had long hoped to find and raise a family. I said to myself, *I must find this valley and return someday.*

I turned back toward the seat in front of me then glanced out again, more determined now to pinpoint our location before the moment passed. At 400 miles per hour, I knew there were only seconds before we moved on. I scanned the landscape for clues and suddenly spotted a building perched near the top of one of the mountains. Bald Mountain? My eyes traced down the slope, following the outline of a town and then, unmistakably, the river bending south through the valley.

To my stunned surprise, it was the Big Wood River—the very river that flows past our home. This was the valley we had already chosen. My wife, my daughter, and our home were already there. The plane had begun its descent en route to Boise. It all made sense now: I wasn't imagining our paradise—I was returning to it.

***

Coming home meant more than just touching down in a familiar place—I was now a father, learning how to navigate a role that was both exhilarating and humbling. Back home, it wasn't that I was a passive or uninterested father—far from it. I wanted to have a handle on diaper bags, baby powder, and the thousand other little things involved in parenting. But I knew where my strengths lay and played to them the best I could. Being steadfast was one of those assets I relied on, and I quickly found myself on night duty. This wasn't a role I had anticipated, but it was one I grew to take pride in. Peggy would prepare a bottle of formula, so I could take over the feedings in the dead of night. My eyes and mind were half-closed as I cradled Blair in my arms. The quiet hum of the house was interrupted only by the sound of her sucking the bottle, the stillness broken only by an occasional cry when she was colicky or when I didn't hold the bottle properly.

While I was good in a pinch, I wasn't the house-husband type and never would be. Interestingly, my younger brother must have inherited the same natural parenting instincts that Peggy had. It clearly skipped over me and went to him, but that wasn't my path—not by a long shot. I had my projects and work to do to support our growing family as best I could. I was as good at real estate development as Peggy was at motherhood. You play to your strengths in a marriage.

New parents often experience necessary isolation. It's not like we wrapped up Blair and took her on a sled dog run around Tin Cup. As young adults whose focus had been on the outside world of adventure and socialization, we turned inward. This wasn't only because Blair had become the center of our universe, though the first year of our firstborn's life was a blur of sleepless nights and long days filled with new responsibilities. Yet, it was also a time when I started reconnecting with myself, trying to find my footing as I juggled the demands of starting a family. Having a child quickly magnifies any cracks you might have in a relationship. Peggy and I didn't have any *Titanic*-sized leaks in the boat, but there were things we had to iron out.

There was a specific time when a heated discussion broke out over whether everything we fed the baby had to be organic. Peggy was adamant: no pesticides, no preservatives, no compromises. I, on the other hand, had just microwaved a non-organic jar of mashed something and thought, *What's the harm?*

Peggy stood in the kitchen, holding the jar in one hand and pointing to the ingredients label, eyes flaring with frustration. "Do you even *care* what goes into her body?" she snapped. Of course, I did. But I hadn't considered going to the same extreme.

Growth is inevitable when you become a parent, as is change. The baby talk coos and gurgles start turning into words and sentences. Then, the little ones can tell you what they want for lunch. Once Blair settled into life and became manageable, I started finding my way in the world again—working, volunteering, and getting involved in everything I could. The work component was a necessity.

***

Just when I thought things around the home had settled down and I had everything figured out, life evolved again. Hayden came in 2000, followed by Wilson in 2003. Hayden was named after Peggy's "partner in crime" from Chicago, Diana Hayden. Wilson was similarly named after Peggy's friend Justine Wilson, who, not by coincidence, is also his godmother. Most people think we named him after the volleyball in *Cast Away*. There's only a small bit of truth there. Either way, I got my boys! As someone raised alongside two brothers, there was something comforting and full circle about bringing sons into our home.

Blair, still so young herself, quickly stepped into a role beyond her years. She was helpful and nurturing, often reminding me of Peggy's meticulous instructions. She was quietly setting the bar for her younger brothers. All three of our children were born in Sun Valley, Blair and Hayden at the old St. Moritz hospital and Wilson at the new St. Luke's facility just south of town. It's still amazing to me to think that these three lives were brought into the world in the small town of Sun Valley, in the heart of a mountain paradise.

John Baker

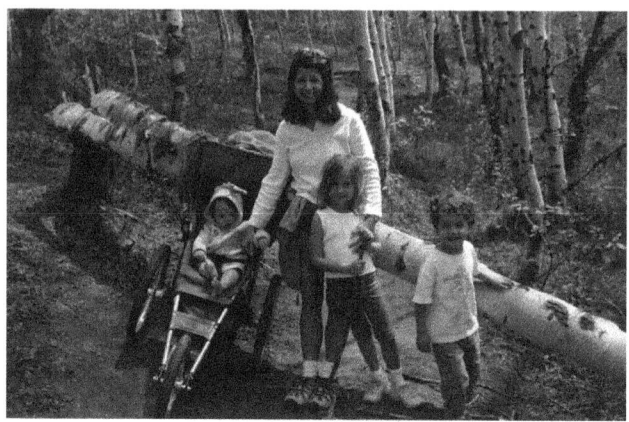

Early years in Sun Valley hiking with the young kids, 2004—
also, the first digital picture stored in my iPhoto library

But now, the cracks in the boat Peggy and I had seen when Blair was an infant seemed to multiply exponentially with Hayden and Wilson on the scene. You'd think the experience we gained from the first child would make rearing the second and third easier. That is true from a technical standpoint, but to use a football analogy, going from man-to-man to zone defense isn't a simple transition.

The real challenges aren't 3:00 a.m. feedings, though. They're the inexorable changes in lifestyle that multiple children bring. I found that parenting three children wasn't the simple joy I'd imagined it would be. My parents and friends who had multiple children had told me that the love I'd receive from my children would make everything worth it. No one ever used the term *eventually* when talking about parenting satisfaction. Looking in the rearview mirror years later, I absolutely agree with my parents and friends and wouldn't give anything up. But at the time, I felt, in many ways, like I was overwhelmed, or as they say in skiing, "over my ski tips."

In Parenting 101, what they didn't tell me was that when you're in the crucible zone, it isn't all cuddles and laughter. The experience, yet again, was nothing like what I had envisioned. As we expanded our family, I felt a strange shift that's hard to describe. I've often likened those early childhood years to running a business with real schedules and deadlines. Not to sound burdensome, but each child becomes another task on an ever-growing to-do list. Even when the to-do list was finished, there was always one more thing. Parenting is never over. Even when the kids are put to bed and you think, *I'm done for the day*, something happens. One of them has a nightmare, needs a drink of water, or wants one more story. It's relentless. The moment you think you've crossed the finish line, out of nowhere, you have another lap to complete. And it's not just the physical tasks—it's the emotional weight, the constant vigilance, the decisions you make knowing they could shape the rest of their lives.

Peggy and I were co-CEOs of Family Incorporated, but the truth was it didn't always feel like an equal partnership. My wife might clarify that she was CEO and Chairman, and I was VP of a small department, mostly taking orders from a boardroom of tiny, irrational executives. And yet, buried under the chaos, there was a quiet sense of purpose—a knowledge that these little moments, the ones that made me want to tear my hair out, were also the ones that defined our family. It wasn't easy, but the most rewarding things never are.

Then, there were the changes in our relationship. Romance took a backseat to logistics. We had to schedule date nights, a concept that felt awkward at first—forced, even—but which became necessary. Even on date nights, it was hard not to talk about something going on with one of the kids. It was like going out with your work buddies and proclaiming, "Okay, we're not going to talk about work tonight!" Then fifteen minutes later, someone busts out a Gantt chart and starts complaining about how incompetent the subcontractors are.

I missed the connection that unscheduled date nights, romance, and, hell, even being goofy together brought. Without those simple connections in place, tensions started to build—at least for me. Peggy was the stable rock, the planner, the one keeping everything together. And me? I was the one who, at times, ran from it all.

Between work and home, there was only so much I could mentally deal with in a day. As our marriage faced more strain, I found solace in work and, of course, the game of golf. A few rounds on the course felt like my escape from the pressures at home. It was my version of breathing room, but Peggy saw right through it. I think on top of being a parenting savant, she's a little psychic, too.

Before our *Titanic* made a beeline into an iceberg, Peggy and I decided to go to marriage counseling. I knew that therapy had helped Peggy in the past, and I was game as long as it would help us figure out where we were going wrong. What I didn't realize at the time was all the problems we had weren't just due to my golf trips or even to slipping off to the golf course during the summer months for a quick eighteen. Peggy was struggling too, and I hadn't been seeing it.

She was a proverbial duck on a lake. Above the surface, Peggy looked calm and in control of everything. Below the surface, she was paddling like hell to stay afloat. My wife was facing the monumental task of raising three kids and keeping a household running. She was exhausted, overwhelmed, and trying to do it all, often feeling like a single parent. Meanwhile, I was out of the house building my businesses and indulging in distractions. We didn't agree on everything, but I'd be lying if I said I didn't see the truth in her frustrations. I had been absent in ways I hadn't fully understood at the time.

Parenting wasn't just hard—it was redefining for me. As we made it through those rocky years and watched our kids grow, I realized that our marriage was changing with us (and thankfully, for the better). Our forged-in-flames relationship came out on the other side stronger. It didn't necessarily happen right away, but our marriage transformed into something more resilient. Our bond became more solid once the kids grew older, once we had less to manage and more to celebrate. I had to remember that phrase I had heard before: "The grass is actually greener where you water it!" In watching the marriages of friends fall apart over the years, I have come to realize this is a super helpful idiom to remember.

Seeing our children grow into young adults, I was proud of who they were becoming—it brought us closer together. And looking back at how much we had overcome, I felt grateful, even proud. Even in the chaos, there were moments—quiet moments—when I would look at Blair, Hayden, or Wilson and see the pure joy in their faces as they came in for a hug or cuddled up for a night time story. These small rewards, these fleeting moments of connection, balanced out the frustrations and made it all worth it.

Heart of the Journey

As for me and kids? It's always been a bit complicated, as I hinted at earlier. It's no secret that I'm more comfortable around adults or even young adults than I am around toddlers or preteens. I've never had the patience or natural ability to soothe a crying child or know precisely what to do when a toddler's temper flares. When I look back, I realize that I probably struggled to understand how children communicate. I wasn't the type to dive deep into the art of baby talk or try to decode every whimper or sigh. But when it came to talking, rationalizing, and discussing things—those were the moments I connected with my kids most. Over time, I realized that I didn't need to be the "perfect parent." No one is. I didn't need to live up to some impossible standard or even be the same parent Peggy was. I learned to become my own type of parent, one who was there when it mattered and supported them, no matter what.

When our kids were of adult age, I remember taking my young nieces, Alice and Sadie, for a short hike around Galena Lodge while my brother was on a mountain bike ride. They were probably six and eight, and I thought I could handle them just fine. I learned from my own kids, after all—what could go wrong? Then my nieces started bickering. One of the girls was calling the other names until she burst into tears. I was lost. I had no idea how to handle the situation. I tried not to lose my cool while diffusing the situation. My solution was rationally saying, "Girls, settle down now, and be nice to each other." The truth was, I didn't have the tools to manage it. It was a humbling experience, and it made me realize that maybe I wasn't as well-equipped as I thought I was or had just forgotten what little skills I once had.

I also know this: Everything I learned, everything I didn't understand, and everything I experienced as a father has shaped me. And I'm still learning. Maybe that's the beauty of it all—parenting never stops challenging you, never stops forcing you to grow. I hope when my kids have children of their own, I'll have the patience to single-handedly take on the challenge, soothe a temper tantrum, and diffuse bickering, to look at myself and say, *I've come a long way.*

27

Family Fun and Fort Maze

How do you want to be remembered?
I want my kids to think I was a good dad.

—Anonymous

While my emotional intelligence with children might have needed tutoring, there were a few things at which I excelled. Play to your strengths, remember? When the kids came along, something else shifted inside me, and it wasn't an avoidance like playing golf. I wanted to share life's wisdom with them as best I could and as was appropriate for their ages. I wanted adventure and activity to be an intrinsic part of my children's lives, like it had been in my childhood. I didn't want them to grow up just hearing stories about the outdoors. I wanted them to feel it in their bones.

I felt this deep need to show them that adventure is not just something you talk about. It's something you live. Making that commitment wasn't easy at first. I was usually coming off a long day at the office or traveling. Honestly, I struggled to transition into "superdad" mode. Peggy was always understanding. She knew that when I got home, I needed a few minutes to shake off the day. But once I had that moment of quiet, I could dive in. Once I found that rhythm, I became better at creating experiences for them, experiences I hoped would become the stuff of family lore.

One of my proudest indoor creations was Fort Maze—a mammoth maze of cardboard boxes that I built during the Christmas holidays, relying on my architectural prowess, carpentry skills, and need for fun. It started small, just a few boxes taped together in the living room, but it quickly snowballed. I suppose it was my way to show the kids that they could be more interested in the boxes than the toys that came in them. Regardless, they loved it—absolutely loved it—and before long, Fort Maze was a full-blown structure that consumed our living space. It had multiple stories, ladders, slides, and secret holes where you could peek out and look down on the world below.

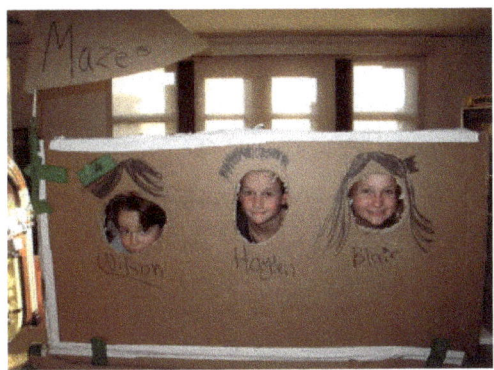

Family fun with Fort Maze

It became a holiday tradition. We'd invite other families with kids over, and everyone would get lost in the maze, giggling and shouting as they discovered new nooks and crannies. Fort Maze wasn't just a physical structure but a metaphor for how we tried to build our family: full of adventure, surprise, and a sense of freedom. One year, it stretched all the way from the upstairs master, down the staircase, and into the living space below. It was truly a maze of slides and tunnels that kept the kids entertained for weeks.

There were other moments in the kids' lives when I got carried away—imagine that. We used to have something I called "tickle time." The kids would pile onto the couch in their pajamas, and I'd chase them around, tickling them until they were gasping for breath. Their laughter echoed through the house, loud enough that I was glad we didn't have close neighbors. It was chaotic, and sometimes, I'd forget that it was bedtime. Peggy would often joke, sometimes with a touch of annoyance in her voice, that I was turning them into hyperactive little monsters right before we needed them to wind down. But for me, there was nothing better than that unbridled joy, that bond we formed through laughter.

When tickle time wasn't an option, we amassed a collection of our favorite books—*The Night I Followed the Dog, Gorp's Dream,* and *Piggy Pie,* to name a few. But the kids' favorite stories were the ones I dreamt up. They were whimsical and sometimes even outlandish stories, and to my surprise, they seemed to love those more than anything we could pull off the shelf. After all, who doesn't like a good story from Daddy? I transported the kids around the world with *The Adventures of the Flying Cow*, *The Talking Dog*, and *A Day in the Life of a Penny*. These stories became multi-night sagas, with the kids eagerly ad-libbing what might happen next.

Though I couldn't be there every hour of every day, I cherished those precious evening moments with their little bodies curled up beside me, as their eyes drooped sleepily and they snuggled into my shoulders. Those were my windows into a quieter kind of fatherhood I hadn't imagined myself being good at. Looking back, it was those moments that began to undo the nagging feeling that I wasn't the most present or proficient dad. The truth was, I was discovering new strengths I hadn't known I had and a deeper emotional presence that surprised me. Maybe I was becoming the father I'd once worried I might never be.

In the winter, we built a mini snowmobile track that wound around the yard—and, of course, the many aerial ski jumps built on the steep hill behind the house offered an element of necessary exhilaration. In the summer, the yard became a place to throw the football, jump on the trampoline, shoot hoops, or take a wedge shot to the golf green I had made in a lower section.

I also realize how much influence our surroundings had on their upbringing. We lived in a ski town, after all. The town and adjacent ski mountain shaped the kids' identities in ways I never fully anticipated. Skiing was a prominent part of that, offering each child a sense of independence.

I started them on Dollar Mountain between my legs, using a harness and edgie wedgies. Then, as they grew more independent, they would meet their friends on the mountain and had the freedom to ski on their own or with the team. Our kids didn't just learn to ski—they became experts. I had been an instructor at one of the best ski schools in the world, after all. When they were old enough, all three of them were cruising down the slopes with ease. They'd eventually go off on their own, enjoying a sense of independence while racing down mountainsides with their friends. I wanted those days to feel like part of the natural rhythm of our lives.

Heart of the Journey

The adventure was never just about nudging them into outdoor sports—though I'll admit, I did hope they'd thrive in those pursuits. For all our efforts to get them outside, I can't pretend it was some picture-perfect experience where we hiked up mountains hand-in-hand, singing in harmony. It wasn't like that at all. There were plenty of times when the kids didn't want to go out on a hike or wake up early to catch first tracks. What we didn't realize at the time was that the example we set for the kids, the quiet way we lived our lives in this outdoor wonderland, would eventually take hold in their minds. We had always thought we were pushing them into athletics. What we hadn't realized was that the pull of the mountains was stronger than any of our efforts. The outdoors soon became as integral to their lives as it was for Peggy and me.

***

The education system in Sun Valley exceeded our expectations. Our children's education began with Montessori school, but as they grew older, they transitioned to the Sun Valley Community School (SVCS), whose outdoor program was second to none. The philosophy at SVCS wasn't just about rigorous academics, though they certainly excelled in that area. The school had something far more valuable: It brought the mountains into the classroom with one of their slogans, "Not All Classrooms Have Walls." SVCS was a gem, founded by a man whose vision combined a college preparatory curriculum with a deep commitment to outdoor education. The students were immersed in the natural world, with each year offering opportunities for real-world experiences. They didn't just study mountains—they climbed them.

The first week of each year at SVCS was always an outdoor bonding trip, where the children could learn survival skills, work together, and test their limits, which I thought were important tools for kids to learn at a young age. My father had wonderful childhood adventures in nature and thought his children should experience the thrill of the outdoors as well. I was now passing the torch to my own children by making sure they had these types of foundational experiences in a safe environment.

The kids had several annual outdoor camping trips, used to strengthen and unify the class. As much as there was resistance to these adventures, they were the backbone of the SVCS experience, proven by the fact that it was what the kids most talked about when reflecting on their time there.

By the time the students became juniors, they were ready for a two-day solo trip surviving on their own in the Utah wilderness. Their final year of high school was showcased by a senior project, wherein they set off for a month traveling and learning about a subject they had a deep interest in. This was a rite of passage where the students took a deep dive into an independent study. I was amazed by how such experiences helped shape our kids into independent, resilient young adults.

It was clear that SVCS's blend of education and adventure was something special. The faculty didn't just teach the kids to excel in the classroom—they taught them to succeed in life. The ski academy, for example, partnered with the Sun Valley Ski Education Foundation. Children could join the local ski team and balance their athletic pursuits with academic achievements. During the winter months, school let out at 1:30 p.m., encouraging all students to get up on the mountain. And then there were the so-called Powder Days—one day each year when the snow was so good that the school shut down to let everyone go skiing with other classes. It felt less like a privilege and more like a cultural tradition, a shared reverence for the snow-capped mountains we called home.

Although my three children attended a school that nurtured their love for the outdoors, it wasn't always smooth sailing. They weren't always eager to join in on every outdoor activity, as I suggested earlier. It was frustrating at first, but then I realized it wasn't about forcing them; it was about setting an example. The culture of Sun Valley, and SVCS for that matter, helped them find their own paths. Some, like Hayden, found their calling in outdoor leadership programs. Others, like Blair, grew into confident and independent individuals in ways I never could have predicted.

When the kids were old enough to understand, I came up with a crafty acronym: RAFT. I had it laminated and pinned to the pantry wall:

R: Respect those around you and respect yourself.
A: Appreciate what you have, not focusing on what you don't.
F: Friends come and go, family is always there for you.
T: Trust in yourself, and be sure others can trust you.

This acronym kept them afloat during their formative years, and I believe it remains with them to this day. What we hadn't fully realized at the time was the surprising and powerful ways our three children were influencing each other. Their sibling relationships were beginning to shape who they were becoming. Alison Gopnik, the developmental psychologist, once wrote, "If parents are the fixed stars in a child's universe—the vaguely understood, distant but constant celestial spheres—siblings are the dazzling, sometimes scorching comets nearby."

I believe now that our children shape each other's choices and life paths not only through natural competition, but also through what psychologists call "spillover effects"—the ripple of one sibling's experiences influencing another's. That idea certainly rings true for me and my two brothers. Wayne, the eldest, chose the stable path of corporate life, drawn to the structure and security it provided. Chris, my junior by four years, found his purpose in teaching—a career defined by the deep reward of guiding others. I, perhaps in response to their choices, gravitated toward a more entrepreneurial route. Where they found comfort in structure, I found energy in risk. Their steadiness may have given me the confidence to take a less traditional path, and in doing so, I carved out a life that felt uniquely mine. In the end, we each took different paths but found purpose in our own ways.

Hayden was working at REI during his senior year of college, and not long after, he headed to New Zealand, where he earned his certification as an outdoor trip leader. During the summer of 2023, he and I ventured on my second climb up Mount Moran, outside Jackson, Wyoming. Hayden and I were roped together at times, having to navigate precarious spots and the tug of the rope. As the rain poured down our first afternoon at base camp, it hit me: There was no better way to bond with your son than being confined to a cramped two-man tent. That is, of course, if you both enjoy the backcountry and don't mind clinging to the side of a mountain.

It felt like a culmination of many things we had envisioned for him, and in some ways, a tribute to my own father for how he and my mother raised me with a love of the outdoors and of adventure. Hayden was a young man finding his path in the wilderness, shaped by the environment in which we'd raised him. I credit my friend, Tim Flaherty, with the idea of including a father–son climb as one of our many adventures. He's an inspirational friend, famous for saying, "I'm in the yes business," especially when it comes to adventure travel.

My daughter Blair had her own pivotal outdoor experiences as well. From a young age, she excelled at figure skating, competing regularly and even performing in front of an audience of 3,000 sports fans during a halftime show. After graduating from high school, she wrote an article for a local magazine about a challenging forty-eight-hour solo trip in the Utah desert—an adventure she was hesitant to take on at first. Years later, Blair looks back on that journey as a defining moment in her life, one where she faced down fear and overcame the challenges nature threw her way.

Then, there's Wilson. He's always had a natural athleticism that I didn't quite possess at his age. One time, he and I ventured to the summit of Mauna Kea on the big island of Hawaii after a rare snowfall. We strapped on skis and carved turns together, making several laps until the 14,000-foot altitude left him a bit lightheaded.

These days, he's retired from ski acrobatics and trampoline flips, trading them in for golf—and he's developed a real passion for swimming and long-distance running. In his own way, he's found his athletic drive, much like I did when I was young.

I can't help but be proud that in some small way, it's the culmination of all those little family moments we spent together that shaped these kids—our adventures, our nights of tickle time, and, of course, Fort Maze. Somehow, life in Sun Valley slowed us down a bit and began to revolve around the towering peaks and sprawling valleys of Idaho. Peggy and I found ourselves immersed in creating a world of adventure for our three children, Blair, Hayden, and Wilson. It was all part of our new life, the one we'd built in a small, ski-obsessed mountain town that embraced the great outdoors in every waking moment.

***

The people and places your children encounter as they grow up are just as influential as the parents who raise them. It truly takes a village. When we chose to live in Sun Valley in 1997—or maybe it chose us—Peggy and I each had our own checklist of "must-haves" in considering various mountain towns. Mine was social: I wanted to be part of a vibrant, tight-knit community of like-minded individuals in a town where you could literally walk to everything. Peggy, on the other hand, was more practical and focused on our future children's education and healthcare. Both were easily found in our growing Community School and our newly built St. Luke's Medical Center. Looking back, it's clear that we'd found the perfect place for both our standards.

Sun Valley has always been where people can shape their identities through the outdoors, though I knew my children might face challenges growing up in a small and relatively homogenous community. Peggy and I were aware of our town's lack of diversity—that's why we believed getting off the proverbial "island" would be crucial for their growth. We tried to expose them to other ways of life and people as often as possible. They met people from all walks of life and embraced different cultures outside our small town.

Along the way, I hoped to instill in them the same core values I was raised with—a love of the outdoors, a strong work ethic, humility, and above all, a grounded approach to life. We wanted to help shape their journey, with Sun Valley as the backdrop. Peggy and I weren't just raising kids; we were raising thoughtful, capable citizens of the world.

We made summer jobs for the kids mandatory, once they were old enough to work. Summer jobs were not a choice, from Leroy's Ice Cream and busing tables at Big Wood Bakery to doing construction labor. This establishment of a work ethic and the value of money at an early age has proven invaluable. Hayden and Blair earned their first paycheck modeling clothing for an L.L. Bean catalog shoot, after a local recruiter in Sun Valley invited them to join.

One day, the kids and I had the chance to sit in a soundproof audio booth with an audiologist, experiencing firsthand the muffled sounds as Peggy hears them. She's worn her hearing aids diligently since Blair was one year old, but her hearing is still far from perfect. That moment deepened the respect she deserves for navigating daily life with such resilience. We wanted our children to be just as adaptable, no matter what challenges they faced.

Our mountain home was a cocoon of sorts, but it didn't hold our children back. They are now out in the world making their paths, excelling in their fields with independence and confidence I couldn't have foreseen. I am incredibly proud that our children moved on to live in big cities like New York, Boston, and London, thriving in environments far from the isolation of Sun Valley.

The outside world might have been unfamiliar to them at first, but they embraced it wholeheartedly. I love our mountain home, and I'm convinced we did the right thing in raising them there, giving them solid roots and the freedom to fly "from here . . . anywhere," which is aptly the motto of the Community School.

I may not have been a perfect father, but I always did my best. I gave my children unforgettable experiences and a sense of adventure. We shared laughter and made memories together. Most importantly, I strived to create a childhood full of wonder for them. They, hopefully, can look back on it with the same joy and nostalgia that I feel when reminiscing about my upbringing. So, next time you're in Sun Valley, surrounded by mountains and maybe even a snowstorm or two, think of us. Our lives may not have been perfect, but they were in the great outdoors together, filled with love, laughter, and some adventure.

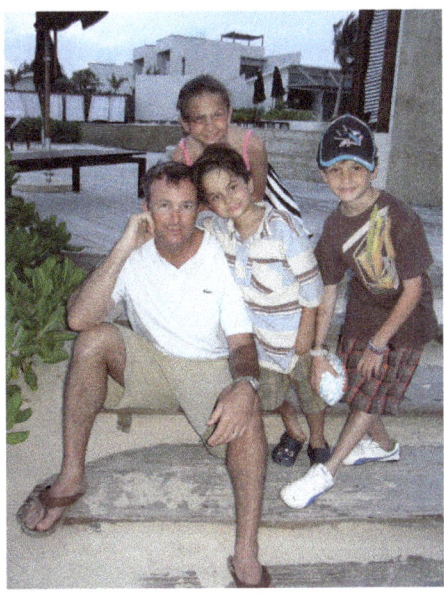

Family vacation in Playa Del Carmen, Mexico

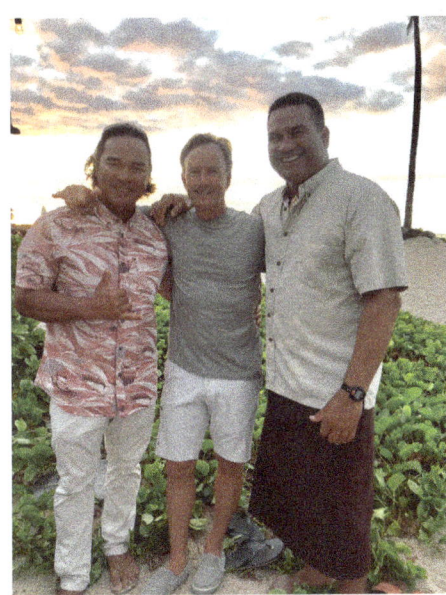

Me with watermen Thibert (left) and Puaita (right)

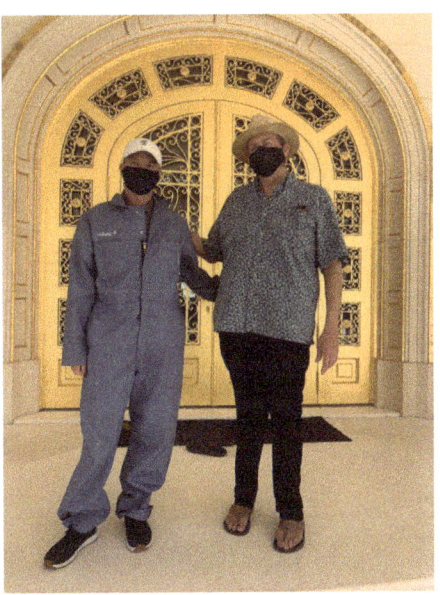

My surprise visit to Andy Mack during COVID, dressed as a service repairman

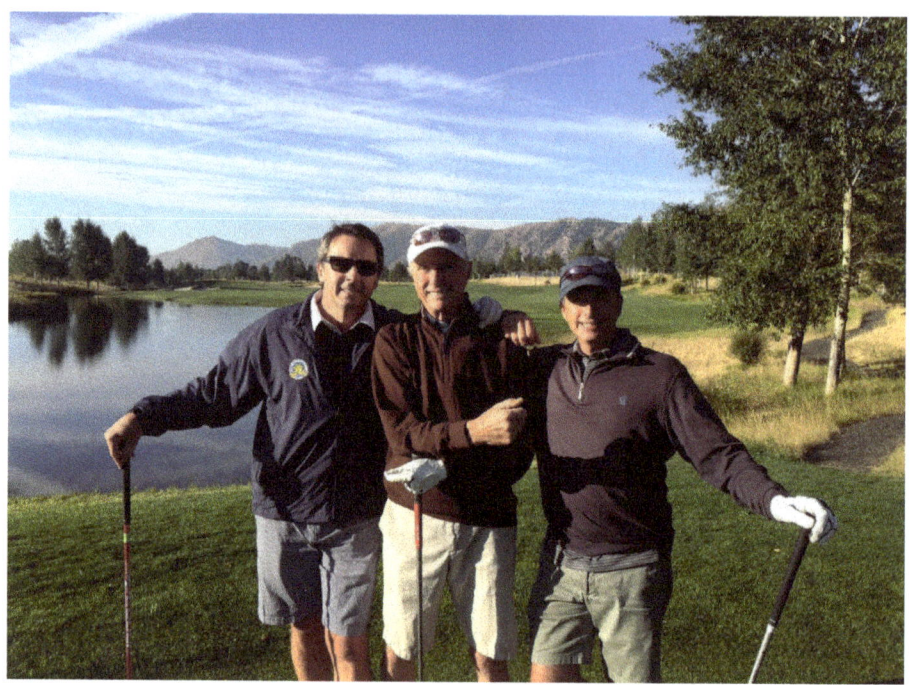
Golfing pals Rob McGowan and Steve Miner

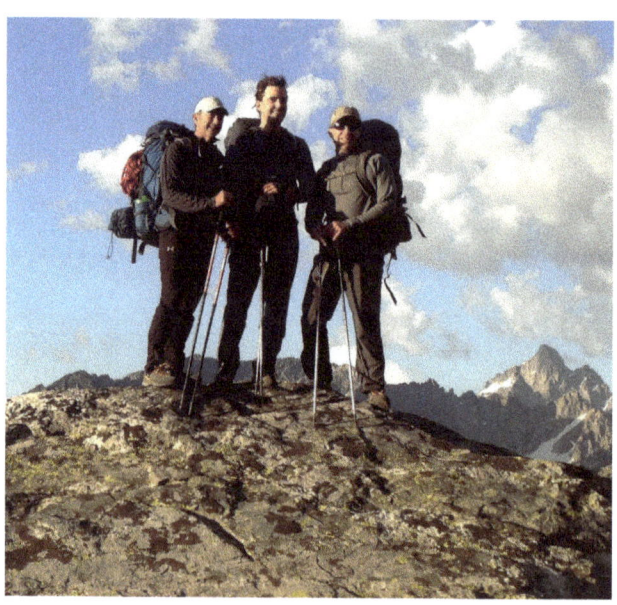
**Me with Thomas Laffont and Doug MacKenzie
at top of Mt. Moran, Wyoming, 2013**

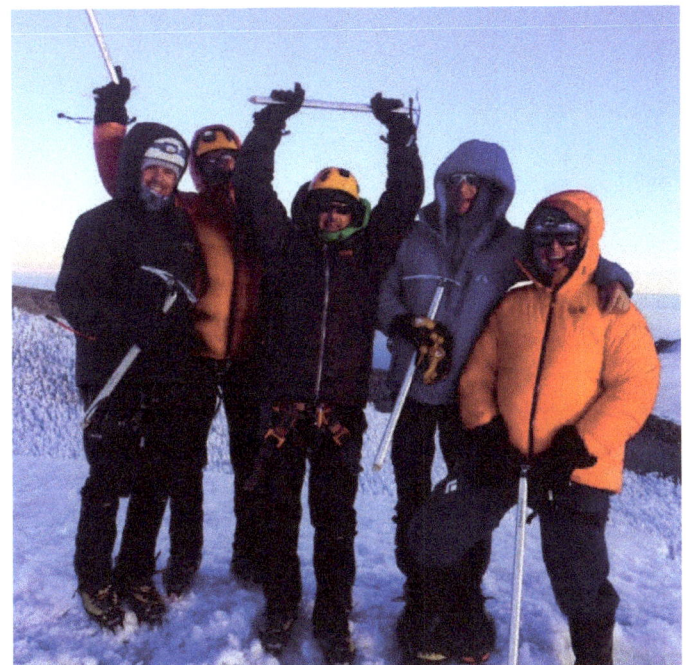

Mt. Rainier, Washington, 2015

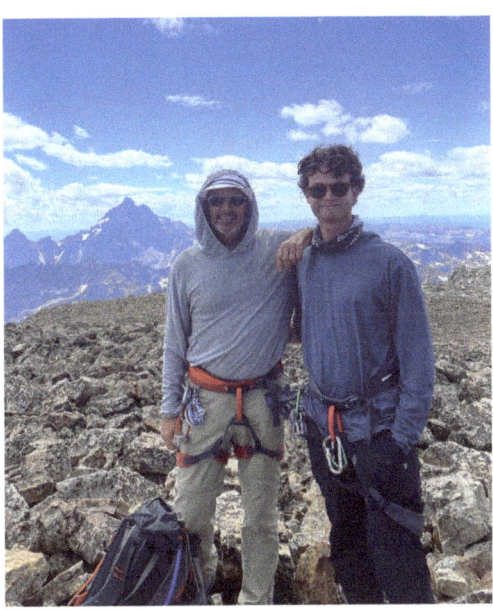

**On the summit of Mt. Moran
in Wyoming with Hayden, 2023**

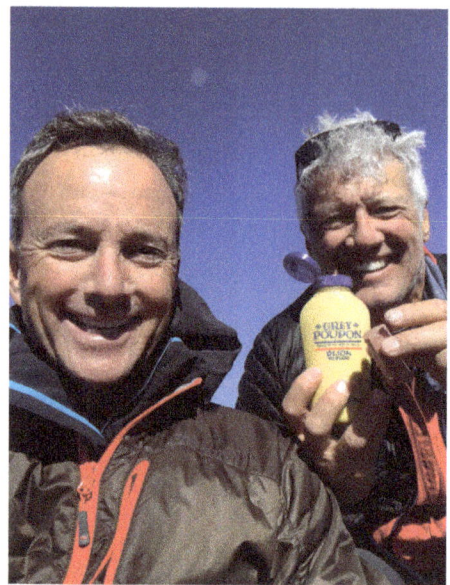

Tradition with Tim Flaherty,
Grey Poupon and salami at each summit,
Mt. Bora, Idaho, September 2018

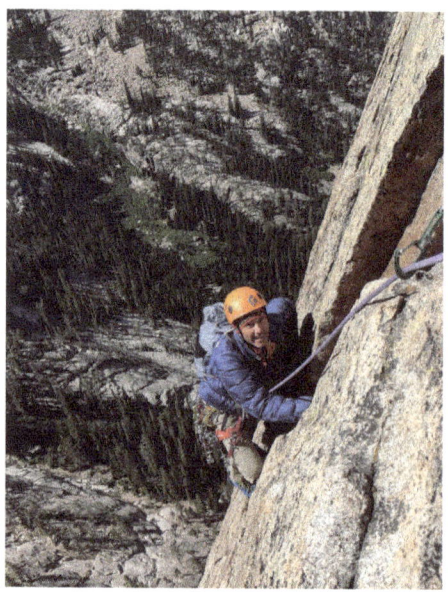

Elephants Perch, September 2017

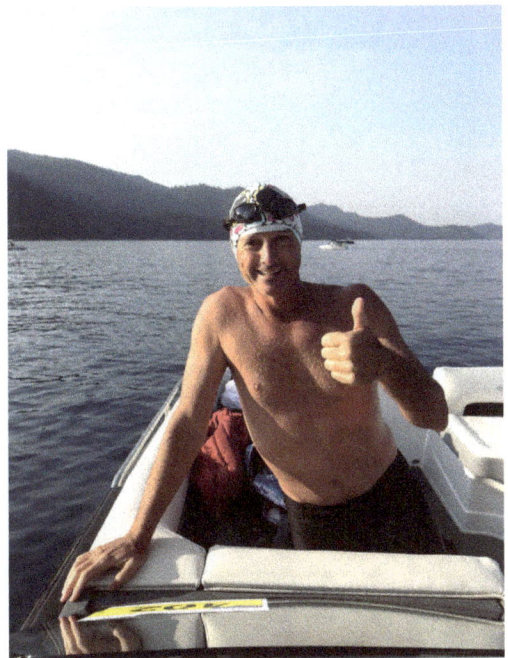

Trans Tahoe Relay, July 2018

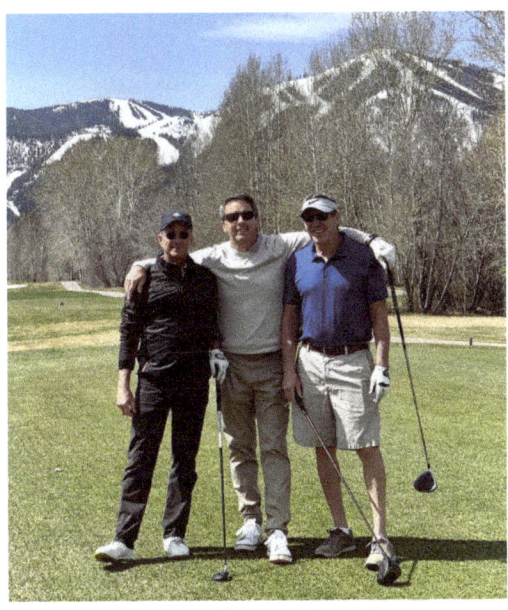

Sun Valley golf with Rob McGowan and Rich Fabiano

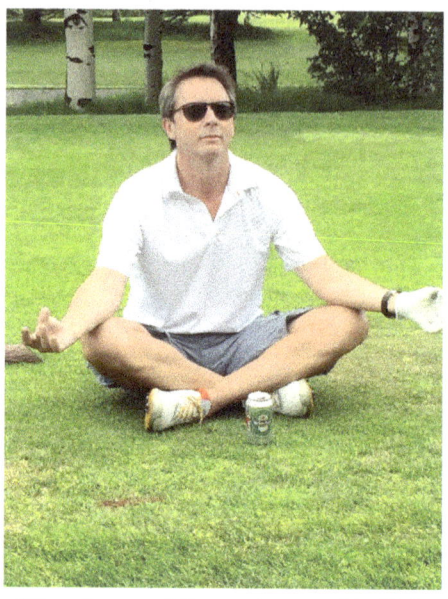

"Serenity now," famously quoted by Rob McGowan at the Valley Club

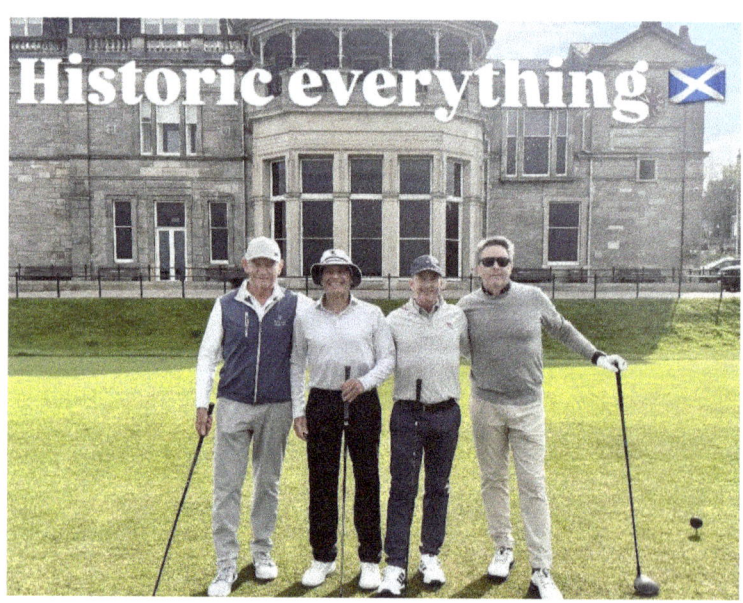

St. Andrews Old Course with pals John Perrenchio, Rob McGowan, and Scott Harris

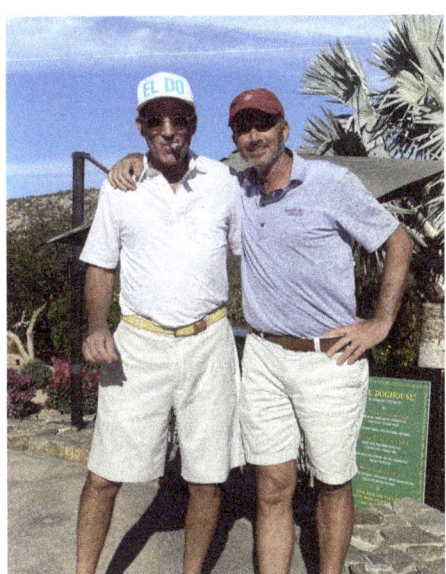

Mike Reynolds needs no introduction

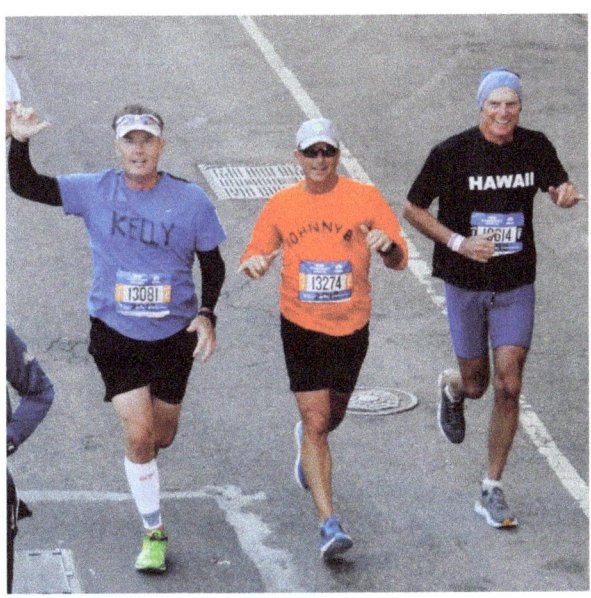

NY Marathon #4 with Kevin Lynch and John Kelly

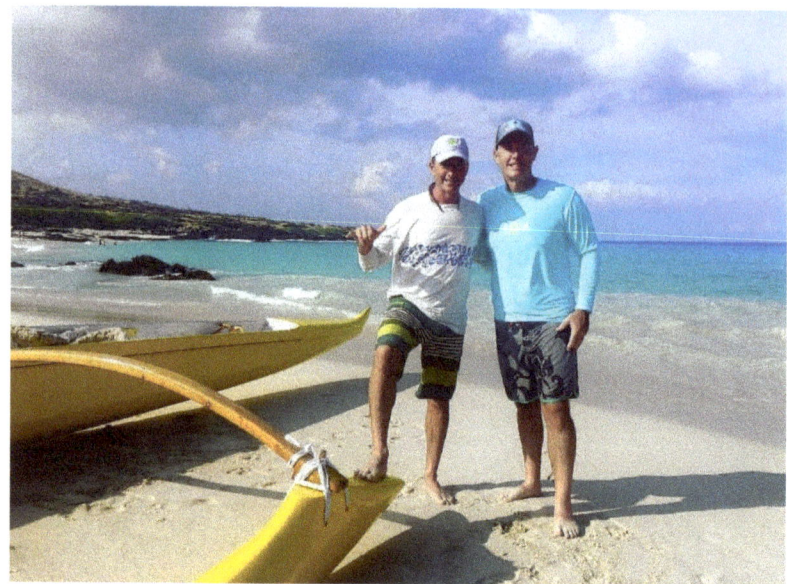

Outriggering with John Kelly in Kona, Hawaii

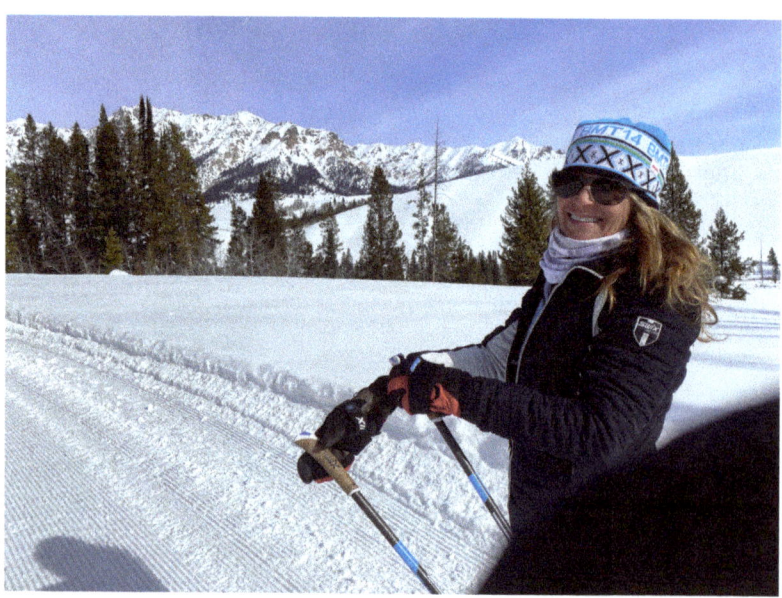

Peggy on the Nordic ski trails, Sun Valley

Heart of the Journey

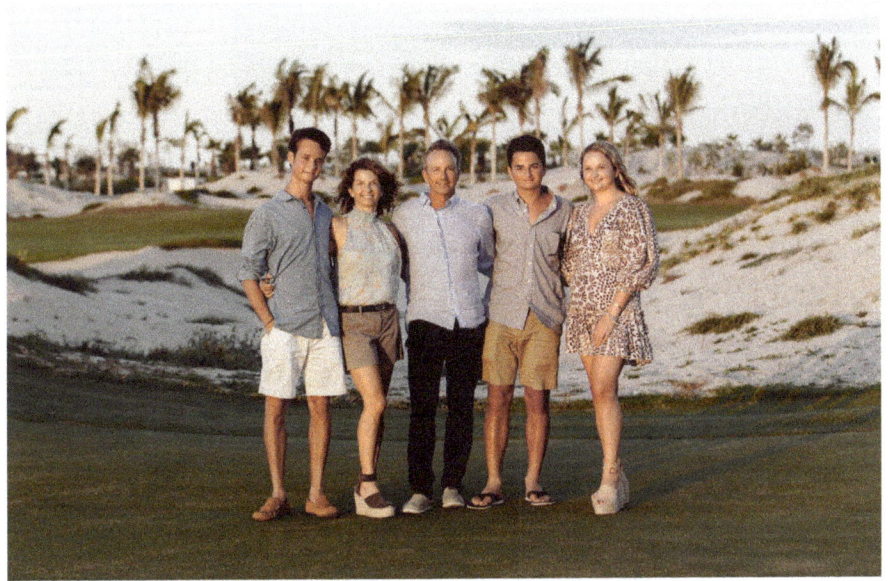

Family vacationing in Costa Palmas, Mexico, July 2020

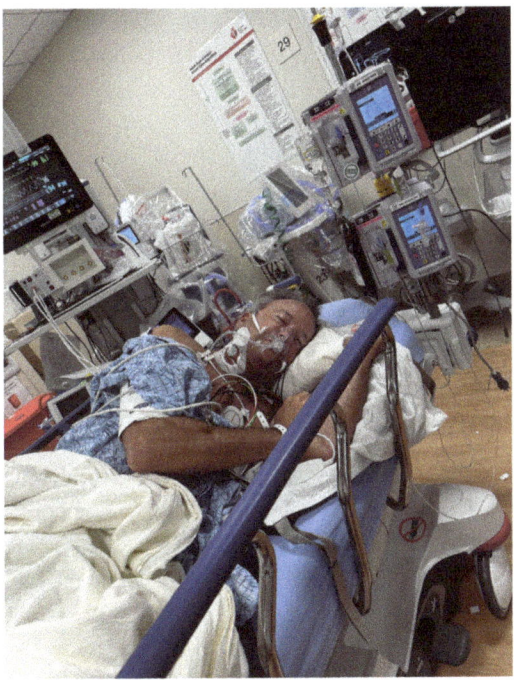

Deep into sepsis shock, April 26th, 2024

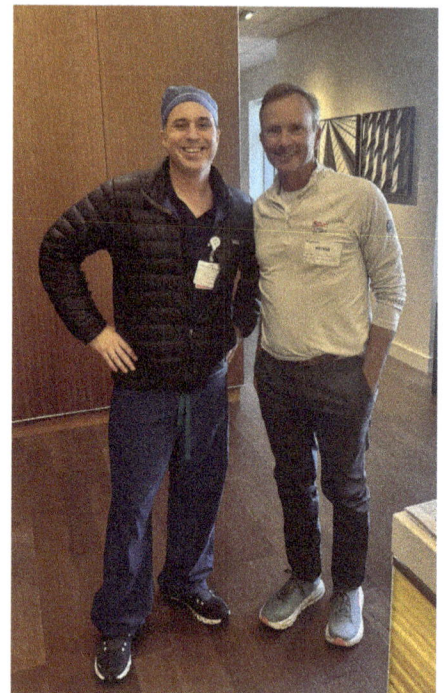

Post-recovery visit with Dr. Daniels

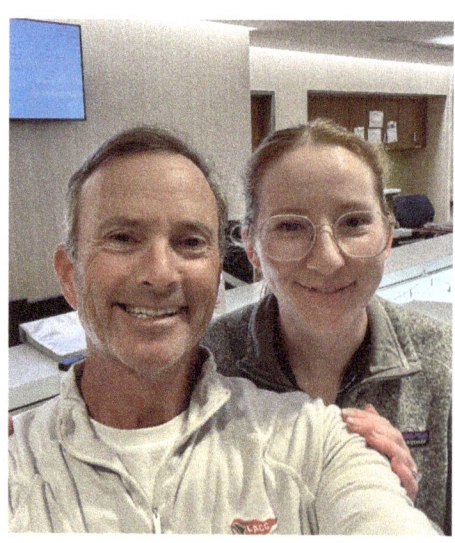

Nurse St. Sophia

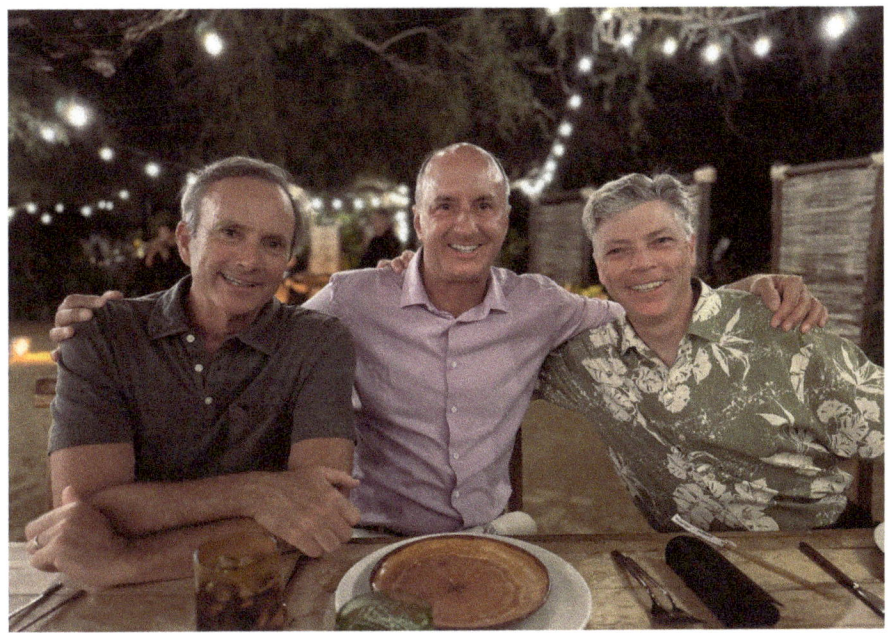

Beau Giannini and Dr. Peter Callander, celebration of health in Mexico, November 2024

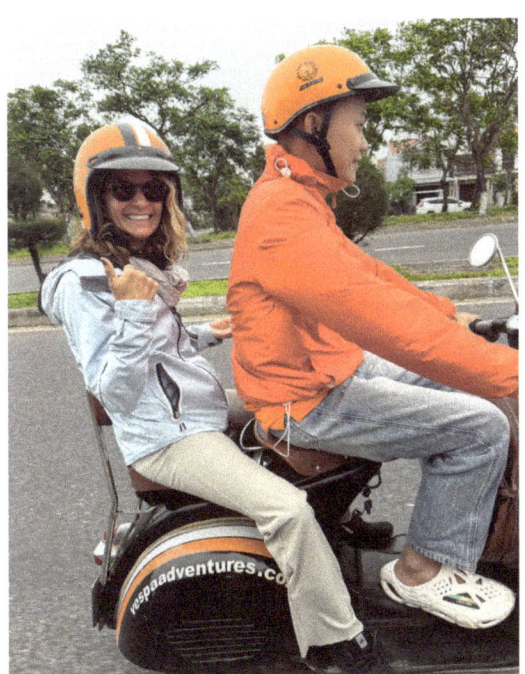

Peggy on Vespa tour in Cambodia, March 2025

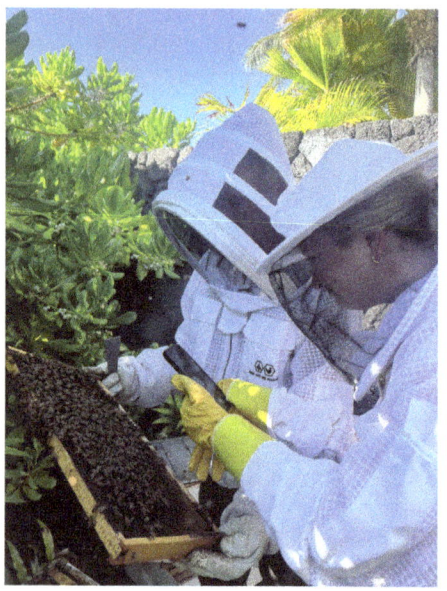
Blair and me, making a hive inspection

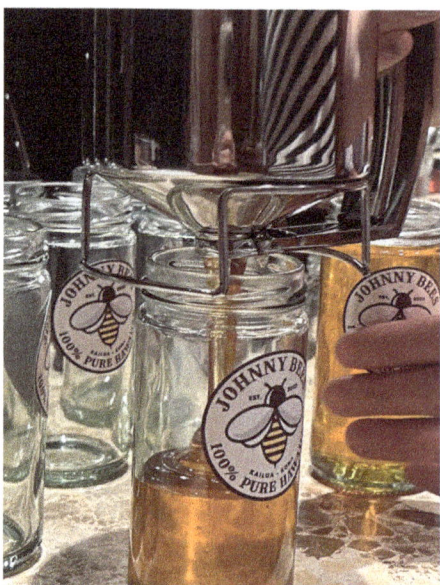
Johnny Bees Honey production

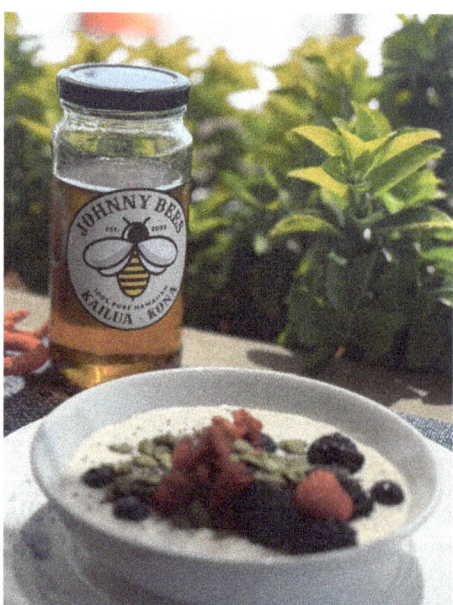
Perfect blend in Hawaii, Johnny Bees Honey

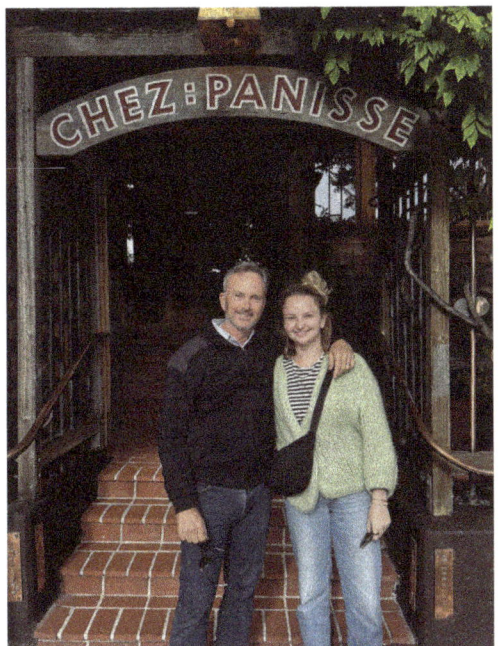

Special moments with Blair, July 2025

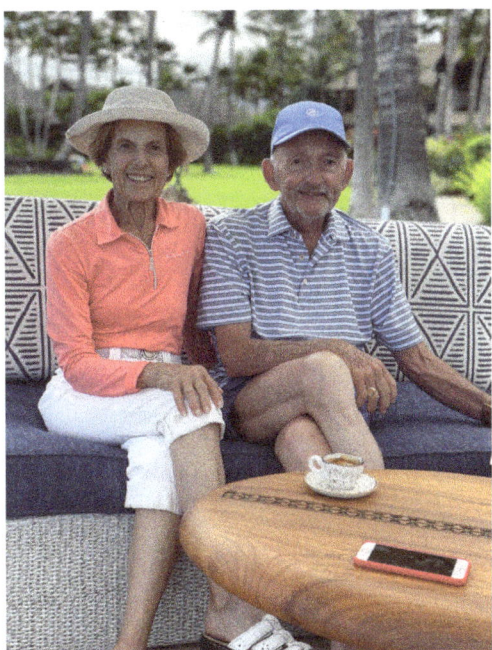

**Bruce and Barbara enjoying Hawaii,
November 2019**

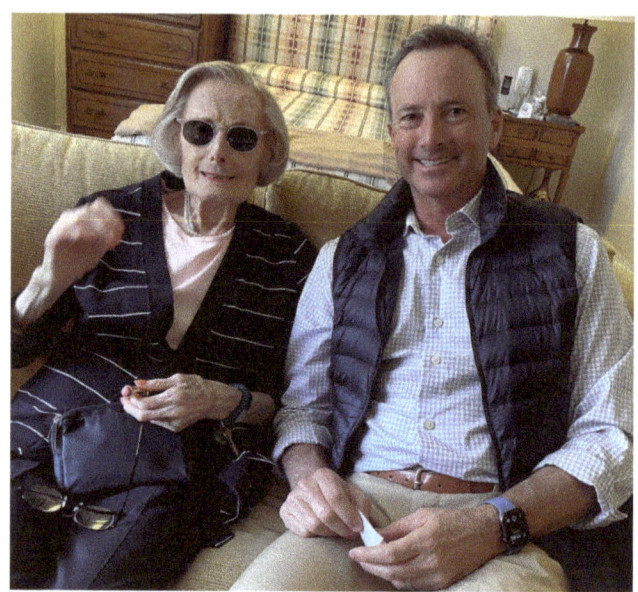

Grandma Terry's apartment, February 2020

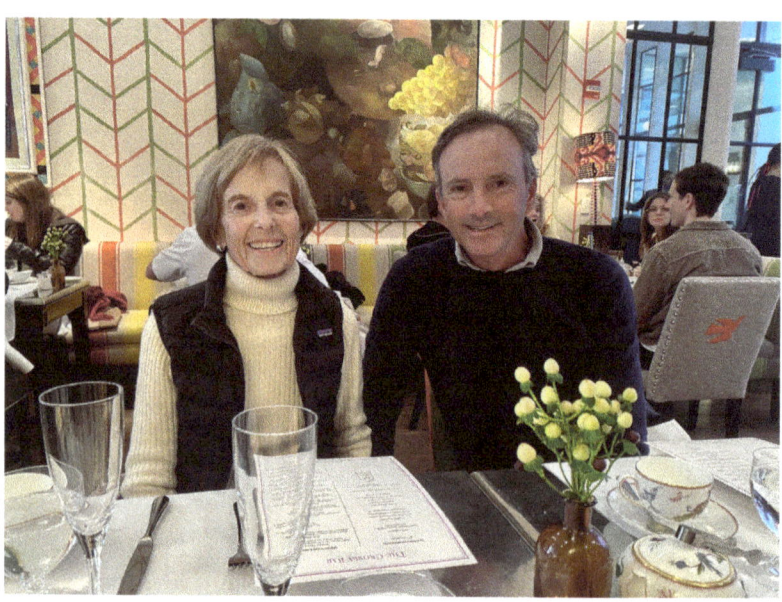

Special time in New York with Mom, February 2024

Heart of the Journey

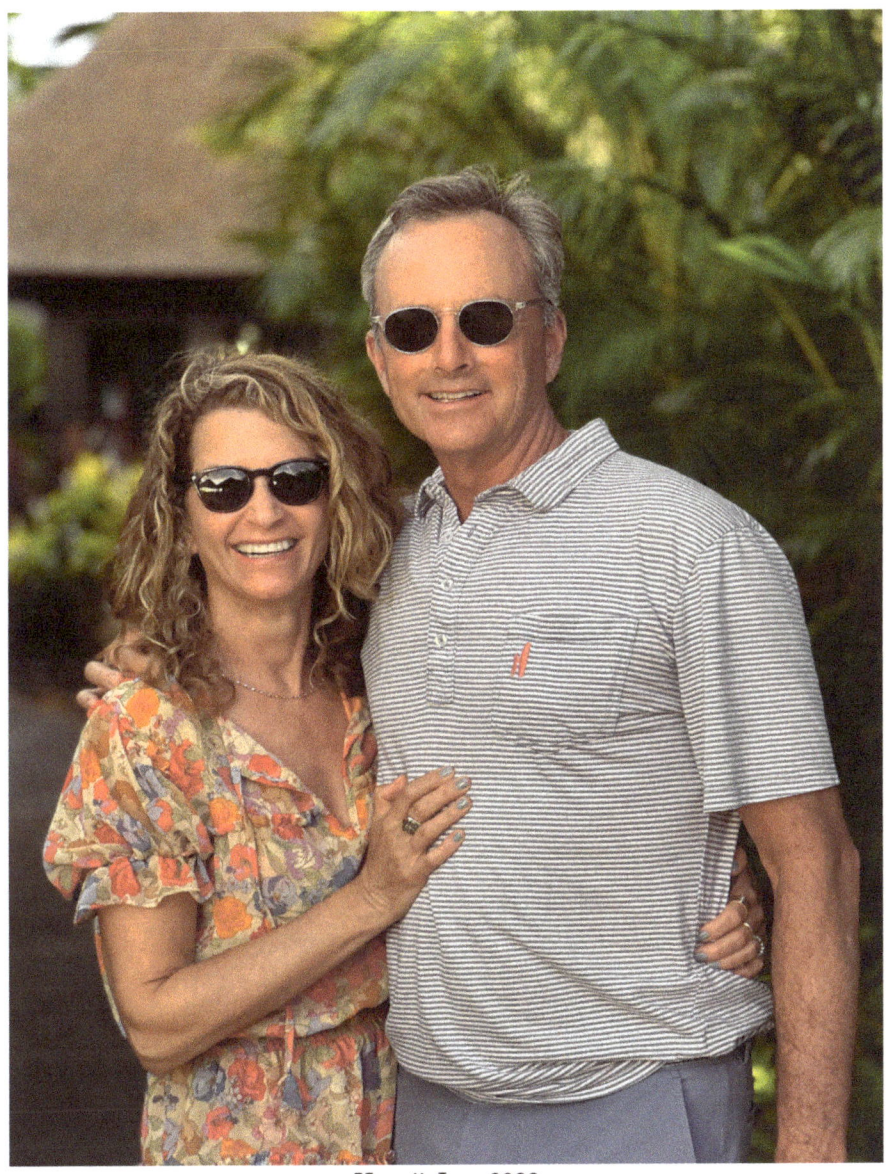

Hawaii, June 2022

28

Career Opportunities

Throw deep.

—Tom Hanks

As Blair, Hayden, and Wilson came into our lives, my career was as much a backdrop to their lives as Sun Valley. Not that this is an excuse, but it was often hard for me to find my footing juggling the responsibilities of husband, father, and businessman. I saw how I fit into the changing dynamic of our marriage through hard work and introspection, and the same happened to me professionally. I didn't realize it then, but every deal I chased and every risk I took would teach me something—not just about business, but about being a father, a husband, and eventually a man who understood when to hold on and when to let go.

When Peggy and I moved to Sun Valley, I was taking a break from construction, adjusting to a new location, and dabbling in several ventures. It was actually the first time we moved for family and not because of a building project. I first started working for a local commercial property owner as the in-house leasing agent. Down the hall from us was something far more exciting and intriguing, a new foreign exchange (FOREX) trading office. I was probably just chasing "shiny things" at this point, but I was drawn to their offering and soon moved my desk down the hall. Over the next several months or so, I learned some of the basics of the foreign exchange currency markets. It opened my eyes to the world of trading that would later come in handy as we started managing our own equity trading accounts.

The following year, I was introduced to two executives in Denver who were capitalizing on the internet boom taking place with Service Magic, a company trying to make the antiquated service provider industry more user-friendly for homeowners. I decided to jump on the bandwagon, working mostly remotely for the company, commuting every other Sunday to Wednesday to their growing home office in Denver. The company was primarily software engineers, plus a few executives who thought they could crack the construction code with a home improvement marketplace. The concept was to create a website that would guide a user through a project like carpeting, cabinetry, or painting by asking a series of multiple-choice questions.

Service Magic needed someone with firsthand knowledge of the industry to create these necessary questions, also called "decision trees," that could generate a cost range and then connect the homeowner with a vetted service provider in their area. It was a unique way to showcase my deep knowledge of the building industry without wearing a tool bag. Back then, I might even have dared to call myself an "industry expert." I disappointed the founders when I chose a salary over private stock options, but it turned out to be the right decision. Though the business is still in existence today under the name HomeAdvisors, it never became mainstream.

In 2001, when Hayden turned one and Blair three, I thought it was high time to get back into the real estate game. I thought combining my GC background, love of architecture, and residential real estate ownership made some sense. I purchased some land in Ketchum on Rocking Horse Way and had a home designed and built. In this case, I wore the title of owner and developer, not architect or general contractor. It was a speculative project, so I assumed all the risk but also reaped all the rewards. I found that I liked being in control of the entire project—top of the heap, from land entitlement through the sale. The Ketchum project worked out nicely, as I sold it during the finishing phases. That allowed the new owner to make a few changes while I secured a nice profit and reduced carrying costs. My plan was simple: Buy land, build an attractive house, and sell it for a profit. It was a modest venture, by industry standards, that brought me modest success, but it taught me about the role of a developer and the kind of risks I was comfortable taking.

The following year in 2002, I rolled some of the proceeds into a lot in a neighborhood in Sun Valley called Elkhorn. I had an architect design and layout an attractive home on the property, maximizing the natural light and grand views. With plans in hand, I started the permitting process. No sooner did someone inquire about the property than they purchased it from me, permit ready.

Armed with the knowledge I had garnered over the past fifteen years—from architecture school to general contracting, speculative building to real estate ownership—I was at a crossroads in the spring of 2002. I knew what to expect when building spec houses. Aside from unavoidable circumstances around market timing, I could make money doing spec work, but the returns were such that I'd always be hustling for the next deal, along with tax consequences from the net realized gains of each sale.

I really enjoyed playing the role of developer, overseeing all aspects of a project, working with contractors and architects, and making the ultimate decisions that counted. I was ready to take things up a notch. This project clarified what I'd sensed for a while: I wasn't cut out to be *just* a general contractor.

There comes a moment when anyone who dreams of creating their own business must take a leap of faith. Whatever that leap may be, it's like stepping off the edge of the pool into the deep end. When any entrepreneur makes that move, it entails a considerable amount of risk and stress. It's a step into the unknown, where the stakes are higher and the safety nets fewer. For me, that leap came over time in the form of larger projects and bigger markets, each demanding more capital, more time, and more faith in my ability to deliver. I often wondered if the risks I took were worth the sacrifices—long days at the office, missed time with the kids, and extensive business travel. I realize now that those challenges weren't just shaping my career. For better and worse, they were shaping me as a husband and father, too. Every deal, every setback, and every triumph taught me something about balance, dedication, and the importance of showing up, not just at work but at home. The lessons I learned on the job—about trust,

Heart of the Journey

commitment, and perseverance—became the same principles I leaned on to build my family and navigate the complexities of fatherhood.

***

I've often been asked why I shifted from residential to commercial real estate development. Both fields shared a similar rhythm—land acquisition, architecture, construction, and occupancy. But I began to realize that the real differences lay in the layers of complexity. In residential development, it's often about time and materials contracts, with room for flexibility and negotiation. Commercial real estate development, on the other hand, is driven by numbers—a world of spreadsheets and schedules, often devoid of the personal connections prevalent in residential work. I saw the appeal of a market that was cleaner, more grounded in market logic, and driven by a formula for return on investment. While spec homes had their value, they were one-offs—passion projects, more art than business.

At the time, I considered advancing into multifamily or larger housing developments in the Boise area. Each property would become a piece of a much larger machine. However, commercial real estate investment was where I decided to focus—office, industrial, and eventually, retail and storage. The market could be unforgiving; there was no sentimentality if a pro forma fell short. If your projections didn't hold, no one would make concessions. Furthermore, tenants would pay what the market dictated, not what my spreadsheet demanded. I'd seen this inflexibility play out. In commercial real estate, any missteps come out of your pocket. No one will sit down for a heart-to-heart if your numbers don't add up.

Commercial real estate is a field with its own set of rules, distinct stakes, and unique sense of freedom. While the risks are significant, they come with the potential for more tangible returns. Cold, hard greenbacks may be a less personal payoff than the satisfaction of creating a home where families will make lasting memories, but there would be room for feeding my soul in the years to come. I was ready to play by the rules and step into a role that made all those years of experience feel like preparation for something much larger.

I realized the common method of syndication was a way to scale up and minimize the risks of larger and more complex projects, but it was a path I wasn't keen to take. Real estate syndications involve pooling funds from multiple investors to collectively purchase and manage larger properties or projects that would be difficult to acquire as an individual. Syndications offer investors passive income potential through rent and property appreciation while sharing the risks and rewards of the venture.

I didn't want to chase large-scale projects involving syndications, excessive fees, and the potential for misaligned partnerships. However, I did want to be in the driver's seat, maintain control, and limit the complications around partnerships. I saw too many peers sprinting toward bigger projects without pausing to assess whether the risk and headaches matched the reward. I wanted to secure a comfortable life for my growing family, but I had to be strategic about it. That wasn't simply a statement about control and risk. I had to also figure out what fulfilled me.

I knew I thrived in a collaborative environment, but I always required a higher level of control and the freedom to answer to no one. Sitting in a room with other professionals and discussing a project was where I felt most comfortable. Each person brings their own unique perspective and experience to the table.

If I followed that vision, syndicated real estate would be out of the question. Knowing that passive investors often didn't fully understand the underlying deal, I had to go a different route, which meant a bit more calculated risk of my own capital. But, if managed properly, this would create far greater rewards. My friend, office neighbor, and real estate advocate, Tim Wolff, would often ask, "So, how much of that capital stack do you hold?" With years more experience than I had, he became the voice of reason, ensuring I wasn't shouldering too much risk.

I also wasn't the idealistic architect Howard Roark from Ayn Rand's *The Fountainhead*. Roark survived on a steady diet of baked beans and stale bread, because no one wanted to build his futuristic designs. Peggy and I were not fans of baked beans. Unlike Roark, I understood that, in the beginning, I would need to balance practicality with ambition until I had built a steady business to take on projects I was truly passionate about.

In late 2002, while building the spec house in Ketchum, I was introduced to a Boise general contractor named Todd Weltner who had been hired to do some commercial work in Ketchum. I could relate to Todd because of his strong commercial construction background. It dawned on me pretty quickly that he would play my role as general contractor, and I could move up the food chain to developer and commercial real estate investor. This was a defining moment in my career. While I needed his boots-on-the-ground talents, he needed my capital and vision.

Todd introduced me to some key players in Boise. For Idaho, Boise might as well be Manhattan. The city was buzzing with opportunity—it was where deals were done. When I first started in Boise, I often heard of agreements sealed with nothing more than a handshake. It didn't take long for me to learn that "the signature is only as good as the person signing it." Boise wasn't just a bigger pond than Ketchum—it was a proving ground where I could test my ideas and build something lasting. That started with making connections with folks involved in every phase of the construction business: bankers, brokers, engineers, architects, contractors, and dozens of other specialists.

One of the brokers Todd introduced me to showed us various parcels of developable land. At the time, large office space was needed in Boise. I believed we had found the perfect place just outside Boise called Eagle River, a development in, predictably, Eagle, Idaho. The grand entrance to the properties made it feel like you were being welcomed to something extraordinary. As we toured the area, I saw the potential immediately. Each lot was carefully marked out, ready for buyers to pick and choose their piece of this promising business community. I selected the most prominent property available, a prime piece of land overlooking a large pond, and hired the best architect I could find in the Boise area. If I were going to do commercial development here, I would do it right.

Todd introduced me to Andy Erstad, the owner of the well-established, full-service commercial architectural firm Erstad Thornton. Todd participated in every meeting and was in the position to turn the blueprints into reality. We had a team in place for my first speculative two-story commercial project. At 18,155 square feet, it sounded like a lot, and for me, it was. But we believed in the location, design, and demand for premium office space in the rapidly growing community just outside of Boise.

It was a gorgeous building when it was finished, and a proud moment for me, because the risk had been significant. When you build something without a tenant lined up, it is always a gamble; however, once the building was complete, it leased faster than I expected. Within months, it generated steady income and proved that the leap of faith had been worth it. I remember the big opening and the excitement of seeing everyone at the broker open house. I was riding high. That project didn't just succeed; it became the formula and foundation for everything I would build or acquire in my career. This was a monumental step for someone who had no real commercial real estate experience—ground-up construction, speculative, with me at the top of the food chain.

Commercial real estate is like eating potato chips—you can't have just one and stop. To succeed the way I wanted, I had to develop leverageable assets with strong tenants and an acquisition cadence that supplied stabilized cash flow. Not that my early days were this planned out, but with my first commercial project giving me cash flow and a modestly profitable sale several years later, I was able to roll those proceeds to purchase the next deal. That formula eventually evolved into a "build and hold" strategy, allowing me to generate a steady stream of income while also providing the leverage to borrow for the next project. Then, it was wash, rinse, and repeat until I had a perpetual money-making machine.

That quick and dirty explanation of creating a commercial real estate portfolio is an oversimplification, but it's the basic framework of how I decided to operate. It also leaves out the part where commercial real estate is about as risky as swimming in the ocean. Eventually, you're going to get stung by something, but you can minimize the larger portfolio risks by diversifying your holdings and always trying to have some cash on hand.

The trick was learning to trust my instincts and knowing when to green-light something, even though the outcome was never guaranteed. I've always gotten myself into trouble when I didn't trust my inner monologue.

At the time, I wasn't just focused on one thing—I was juggling multiple ventures, each pulling me in a different direction. It was chaotic, exhausting, and exhilarating, like standing in three rivers at once to see which one would carry me furthest. I was traveling frequently, managing my first large-scale real estate projects in Boise while simultaneously launching a sourcing and manufacturing business in Shanghai called Boardman International. That venture was with my longtime friend Beau Giannini, who spoke Mandarin fluently and had relocated with his family to Shanghai, building a sourcing business of his own from the ground up. I was drawn to being in business with Beau, especially one that was capitalizing on the real shift our country was making in globalization.

Most evenings, I'd shift gears and dive into late-night calls with Beau, navigating time zones and language barriers to source medical products for U.S. distribution. Our proudest collaboration was designing a surgical clipper with disposable heads, a product we patented and is still distributed worldwide today. This business continued for three years, when I realized I needed to allow for more family time and to focus on my primary business of real estate. I sold my interest to Beau, who has continued the business to this day.

One of my favorite memories with Beau in China was not on the factory floor, but when we hiked a remote section of the Great Wall together—a four-hour journey along the wall from one small town to another with no other tourists around. Walking that ancient structure with the weight of history beneath our feet, surrounded by Chinese countryside on one side and Manchurian on the other, was simply mind-blowing. But not all of my business adventures at this stage of life were uplifting.

***

One early experience where I bit myself in the ass was another office building opportunity in Eagle River with the owner of the development. When I first met him, we hit it off. He was experienced, well-connected, and eager to work with me after our first Eagle River project was successful and caught his attention.

He was twenty years my senior and a seasoned developer out of Phoenix. Once I'd finished the Eagle River office building, he approached me to say, "Great job! Do you want to do another one?" Coming from someone with his experience, that felt like validation. Then, he offered to partner with me, and I got all moon-eyed, like the prettiest girl in school had asked me to the prom. Here was this big-time developer wanting to team up with me. I thought, *What an opportunity.*

A learning experience would be more like it.

Todd Weltner was yet again the perfect fit for the job. Together with the architect, I reassembled our team to bring this second ambitious vision to life.

The project began in the summer of 2004 and was on track for completion when my partner became unreasonable with our contractor, Todd, attempting to create a rift between him and me. On top of that, we faced significant unforeseen expenses with the city, and things quickly took a turn for the worse. My development partner was livid and thought I was to blame. I don't recall all the details of what he said, but it was stern enough, and the fallout was messy. We finished the building, leased it out, and even added nice touches, like my personal artwork in the common areas—something I took pride in. But my partner had turned on me. At that point, I told him I wanted to dissolve our partnership. He agreed to buy me out, but not without making things as difficult as possible. He refused to pay for the art, nitpicked over expenses, and left me feeling burned.

The silver lining was that I didn't lose money, but the difficult experience left a bad taste in my mouth. To make matters worse, he used the building designs we'd developed as the template for the rest of his development. Suddenly, my vision was replicated all over Eagle River, but without me involved. Ideas aren't like songs. You can't get royalties every time your concept is used the way Led Zeppelin gets a payoff every time "Stairway to Heaven" gets streamed. It stung to see my hard work co-opted, but I learned a valuable lesson: Not everyone in this business is honorable. Just because someone has been in the industry for twenty years doesn't automatically make them a good person or business partner.

Overall, this experience solidified something for me and sharpened my aim. If I were going to have a financial partnership in business, it'd either be a bank or someone I knew and trusted intimately. From then on, I decided to trust my more refined instincts, take control, and minimize the risks of relying on someone else's integrity. It was a painful chapter, but it shaped how I approached the next phase of my career.

29

Deals and Diversification

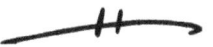

No one cares about your money as much as you do.
—Jim Mills

The funny thing is, I never set out with a roadmap to build a diversified real estate portfolio. It just happened—one deal led to the next, like steppingstones across a fast-moving river, each requiring a little leap of faith. Maybe that's what drew me in from the start. There had always been a sense of adventure in the real estate industry; it wasn't flying down a mountain bike trail or being roped up on a rock face, but it had its own kind of thrill. Each project offered a new landscape, a fresh set of challenges, and that familiar rush of stepping into the unknown—of trusting your instincts and hoping the landing was solid. It scratched the same itch I'd chased in other parts of my life: the drive to challenge myself and build something lasting.

I didn't always have perfect balance, but what I did have was a drive to keep building on the foundation of my architectural background. If Sun Valley gave us a home, my work gave me identity, purpose, and, at times, a sense of control in a life that was becoming increasingly full.

After building the office properties at Eagle River, Shoreline, and Bown Crossing, I found myself caught between two approaches: developing land from the ground up or purchasing existing properties. Development offered a clean slate, but it was a lengthy, highly speculative process—and at times, it didn't sit well with me, especially when I watched a pristine piece of land scraped bare by a bulldozer.

On the contrary, I was especially proud of the 416 S 8th Street property purchase, in a sought-after historic area of Boise known as BODO—Boise Downtown. This corner building was a lofty brick structure with tall ceilings and huge wood timbers, once serving as a warehouse for storage and distribution. I took great pride in preserving its architectural integrity while leasing the building to technology-minded businesses and hip creative types, including Drake Cooper Ad agency.

I had also purchased an existing multitenant retail property at 471 Leadville in Ketchum, previously known as the Crazy Horse Building. While it was easy to manage a smaller property in our valley, it made me realize even more that I needed to be in a larger metropolitan area, where real business transactions with normalized cap rates occurred along with capital appreciation and all the benefits of positive cash flow.

My first steps into geo-diversification came almost accidentally in Palm Desert, California. We started vacationing there as a family in the early 2000s. It was precisely the opposite of living in the mountains in Idaho. The mountain retreat of Sun Valley has crisp alpine air and world-class skiing. Palm Desert, by contrast, is a desert oasis offering warm, sun-soaked winters and lush resort golf courses. We were drawn by the warmth and a craving to escape our everyday surroundings. Inevitably, my curiosity about the local real estate market kicked in. What began as a few exploratory conversations turned into a limited liability holding company called Desert Properties, a company dedicated to a couple of commercial real estate properties in the area.

My first solo project in Palm Desert was The Gallery Building, located on North Palm Canyon Drive. Like the historic property in Boise, it had been repurposed and needed some TLC. It was originally built as an auto garage, with a beautiful wooden vaulted ceiling spanning the interior, and was later repurposed into an office property. It was an architectural gem that, for me, was more than just an investment.

The following year, I partnered with Jim Bishop, the contractor who had built both our homes in Sun Valley and the spec home on Rocking

Horse several years earlier. We purchased a strategically placed industrial parcel of land on Leopard Way in Palm Desert and built a concrete tilt-up, multitenant industrial building. The industrial market was fairly strong, so we had little problem leasing it and creating some nice cash flow. These properties were manageable and offered us not only good real estate experience but an excuse to travel to the warm desert with my young family. Jim brought the expertise and some capital, and I managed the project. Peggy's mother, Dorothy, believed in me early on and lent some of the equity for the project, along with the Gallery Building property. When the 2008 financial crisis hit, Jim's business took a hit, and he asked that I buy him out. That experience taught me the value of liquidity and having the means to weather bad times.

***

The 2008 financial crisis was obviously a challenging time for real estate in general; however, interest rates, and therefore borrowing costs, were substantially reduced, spurring low interest rate borrowing for those that were qualified. At the time, Peggy and I had switched to a different financial advisor at RBC Dain Rauscher. While the relationship only lasted about three years, the advisor did a few things right: He helped to negotiate borrowing with Fidelity Investments at 25 basis points (0.25%) over Fed funds. In effect, I was borrowing for less than 2% during the real growth years of my business. As our wealth grew, it was a luxury to borrow this way on a shorter-term basis, though I still utilized the local and regional banks for securing longer-term loans.

Back in Boise, I dabbled in a group of multitenant industrial properties called Stratford Industrial Properties, a far cry from the office buildings. These were 15,000 square feet each, so quite larger than the Palm Desert industrial property. They were straightforward, tilt-up concrete utilitarian spaces where function trumped form. With my architectural background, I was surprised that I found interest in industrial spaces; however, if I were to continue growing, I needed to consider them. Further, they required less management due to the nature of their triple net leasing. Basically, rent is collected with the landlord/owner only needing to take care of the building structure.

My Boise broker, Shane Jimenez, was actively showing me other properties in the area and started investing some equity alongside mine. Even though they were minority stakes, it meant our interests were aligned; he would only show me properties that made financial sense to him as well. We continued acquiring in the Boise area over the next few years with a stand-alone Starbucks and drive-through, several sprawling self-storage facilities, and Eagle Storage Condos. It was a niche storage sector I hadn't even known existed when I first got into the game.

These huge units, sold individually, are the types of storage areas you typically can't build at home. They house all the large toys for the outdoorsman and hobbyist or make for perfect workshops and spaces for small distributors. This concept of a storage unit for ownership has been a great product offering. I really enjoyed the product mix of traditional self-storage and the concept of allowing ownership of larger units in our storage condos. I've said many times that if I could go back in time, I would have just focused on the self-storage industry. It's such a unique product in the world of real estate.

All these properties and the land I purchased for future development taught me over the years how to operate a successful real estate business, including negotiating lending terms, leases and contracts, entitlements, tenant improvements, property management, and partnerships (the good ones and the bad). It was never just about square footage or rental income—not really. For me, each property had a pulse. A new building meant solving a puzzle, making a dozen judgment calls a day, and watching something physical rise from nothing. I loved that and still do. But over time, I began to see that what I was really building was *experience*—and slowly, something that looked like a life I could be proud of.

Another turning point occurred in 2011, when Peggy and I woke up to the fact that we needed to think about managing our own money outside of real estate. We decided to remove our financial advisor and started managing our own stock investment accounts. Many of her family members were already doing this, so we took the plunge. I learned over time that the advisor's first allegiance is to himself and his family (as it should be), then to the financial institution where he hangs his hat, and finally to the client.

We flew to Chicago to meet with Peggy's father at his office to learn about trading the options market. This was a pivotal time in learning to take full responsibility and accountability for our investments. It wasn't easy going "back to school," but we studied independently, and over the course of several months, we started to research specific stock positions and characteristics to carefully execute small options trades. I recall Peggy and I hitting the "trade" button for the first time and then calling her father to make sure we understood what we had done.

I still have documentation of the actual trade:

CALL (AAPL) APPLE INC FEB 18 2012 $420 (100 SHS) 5 contracts

The value in options trading has been tremendous. It forced us to understand the underlying stock assets and has increased our overall annual market returns constantly by 1–2 percent. Most importantly, it has given each of us investment roles: I do the research, manage the underlying stocks, and advise on which should be optioned, while Peggy researches the best strategies and executes all trades. We don't sit across from each other, because even hearing the tapping of each other's keyboards often annoys us. We do, however, work on our own schedules and use email to document all communication around trades. Since we began trading together in 2012, neither of us has disrespected the other one's decisions—quite the contrary, in fact. We have grown to respect each other's discipline, even if our approaches sometimes differ. That's not to say we haven't had to make difficult decisions or strategize the best way out of specific trades. But we let mutual respect guide us, which is certainly good practice for any relationship.

Whether trading in the stock markets or managing an office property or self-storage facility, the game was always about balancing the potential for reward against the possibility of being stuck with a nonperforming or declining asset. In real estate, I might have diversified a little too much at times. Each sector and location brought its own set of challenges, and the headaches that came with juggling such a wide array of investments in differing markets took a good team in place to properly manage. But back then, I thought the broader my portfolio, the better my odds.

It was around this time a friend of mine named Reamy Goodwin asked me over lunch, "So, how's the real estate empire, John?" While it was far from an "empire," I was proud of all the transactions and successes and knew it was adding up. I enjoyed most aspects of the industry—specifically, the pride of ownership.

30

Quiet Chaos

You keep running, you don't quit, because when you add up all those accomplishments and silly things, what they add up to is . . . your life.
—Casey Neistat

In those early years, there was a quiet kind of chaos to juggling multiple developments. But I didn't stop investing when new opportunities came knocking—I expanded. The timeline of my career became an intricate web of overlapping ventures. By 2014, I was continuing to venture out of the Boise market. That year marked a turning point not just in geography but in how I approached the tools I needed to keep my business agile.

That's when I bought the plane.

Now, let me be clear: When people hear you own an airplane, they picture something extravagant, with flight attendants asking, "Mr. Baker, can I get you a glass of champagne?" The Pilatus PC-12 wasn't a flashy airplane. The aircraft was a single-engine workhorse that could land on short runways, ideal for the mountainous West. The aircraft seated eight comfortably and is endearingly known as a Suburban with wings. I managed it through Western Aviation in Boise and integrated it into their charter program. The idea was simple: I would outfit it with in-demand Wi-Fi, a rarity for small planes back then, and let the business community put it to use.

The aircraft's setup was more pragmatic than indulgent. There was a cash outlay up front, but the charter income offset most operational expenses, and the write-offs kept my accountant happy. It's not something I'll ever put on record as profitable, but it certainly paid for itself. That plane symbolized something greater than convenience: flexibility. For five years, it allowed me to navigate a growing portfolio of developments while maintaining a foothold in the Boise area.

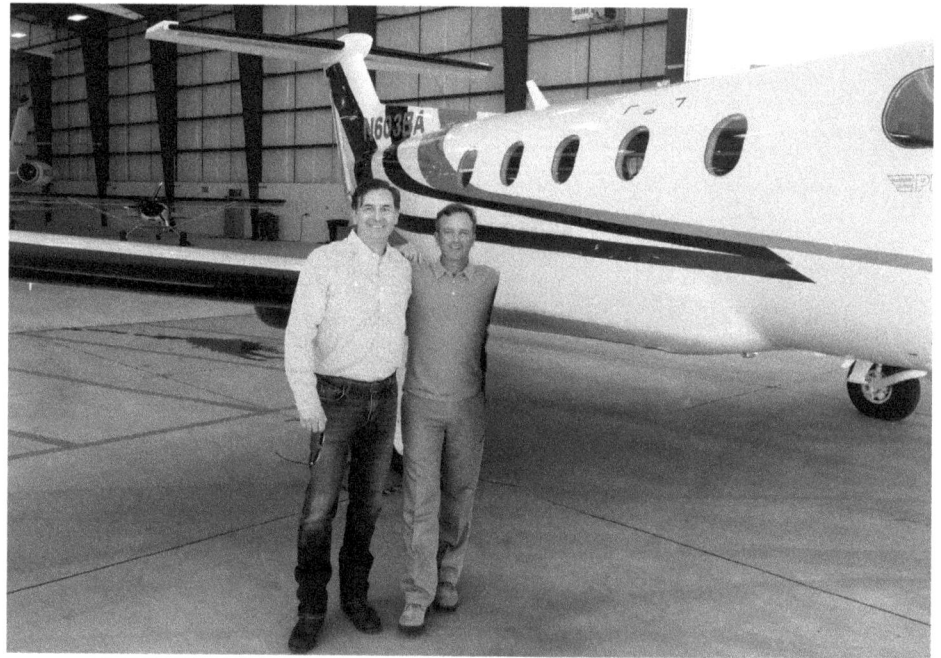

Shane Jimenez and the Pilatus PC-12

More importantly, the aircraft represented the ideological shift in my business I'd been searching for. It was no longer about grinding out every cent of margin or clinging to every project with a white-knuckled grip. The plane embodied leverage—the ability to delegate, expand, and think bigger without sacrificing my time or health. The aircraft was freedom, not just in movement but in mindset. I had a tool that allowed me to scale up my business without worrying about the hassles of travel. For the first time, I wasn't chasing my business—I was steering it.

There had always been a sense of adventure in this industry that I genuinely enjoyed, something that reminded me of other risks I'd taken in life. Just like the mountains I'd climbed or marathons I'd run, each deal came with its own terrain, its own weather, and its own kind of thrill. Real estate may not seem like a wild ride from the outside, but for me, it scratched that same itch of stepping into the unknown with patience and conviction.

Taking control meant developing a strategic vision for my business interests that went beyond just looking for the next deal. I needed to diversify my holdings while focusing on a few geographically strategic areas. With the help of Shane, we decided to expand our Boise portfolio outside Treasure Valley and into the Pacific Northwest—specifically, to a large retail complex in Bonney Lake, Washington, outside Seattle, called The Market at Lake Tapps. This sprawling retail center also included out-parcels with a car wash, a bank, a Jack in the Box, and a Starbucks with drive-through.

It was at this time when I said to the brokerage team, "If this purchase price is that good, then you should be putting all of your brokerage fees into the deal." Sure enough, that's exactly what they did. We continued our acquisitions with two other neighborhood center complexes, one called Westpark in Billings, Montana, and the other called Chandler Heights Marketplace, outside Phoenix, Arizona. These years taught me that diversification was more than practical—it was essential to creating a successful business. The lead broker, Shane Jimenez, remains a broker, asset manager, business partner, and friend to this day.

I always liked to use the word *we* when discussing my properties. Even though I was the managing partner and usually held north of 90 percent ownership, I believed it offered respect to the brokers and smaller investors that came in along the way. Additionally, if you think of investments as a percentage of wealth, the dollar amount didn't matter: It was a percentage of that individual's net wealth, so it meant as much to them as my investment did to me.

I feel compelled to share the most frustrating borrowing experience of my career—not because of the numbers, but because of what it revealed about the system I was operating in. It was a commercial mortgage-backed security (CMBS) loan that I'd assumed from the previous owner of The Market at Lake Tapps. On paper, it looked attractive: lower interest rates and non-recourse terms. But the reality was anything but.

The loan had been bundled with others and sold off, managed not by a bank but by a loan servicer—an anonymous entity with rigid demands and no meaningful interest in the long-term health of the property. Their requirements were excessive: They withheld a full year's worth of insurance, taxes, and maintenance costs in escrow, as if I couldn't be trusted to pay them myself. It wasn't just inefficient—it felt punitive. The retainage drained cash flow, limited our ability to maintain the property well, and created a relationship built on suspicion, not partnership. Looking back, it was an early sign that my frustration with the industry was beginning to surface—one of the first cracks in my lifelong career of real estate investment.

***

You never really know when stocks will rise or fall; the same goes for real estate. Market crashes, tenant departures, and unforeseen disruptions are part of the game, but success hinges on staying power and creative restructuring when necessary, both financially and mentally. I learned this the hard way when I lost an anchor tenant—and with them, millions in future rent. Lucky's Market, a Kroger subsidiary, filed for bankruptcy and walked away from a lease on a property in Billings, Montana. Kroger itself wasn't going under; in fact, they had more than enough capital to honor the leases. The lawyers just decided to use the crafty bankruptcy laws to move the burden onto the property owner. It was a calculated move that left me furious. Over ten years, that lease would've been a significant income stream, but suddenly, it was gone. The experience taught me that resilience and a long-term perspective are critical, because you never really know when you might lose a valuable tenant.

But that's the game. If you have the staying power, you can time the market right on your way out. That's the formula that's worked for me: Buy smart, hold steady, and sell strategically. Looking back, I never aimed for home runs. Base hits have always been enough as long as they added up. For me, success has also been less about contracts and more about the people behind them. Deals are only as good as the trust between the parties involved. I've been fortunate to work with some of the best.

Surviving the financial crisis of 2007–2008 made me feel somewhat bulletproof in the real estate market, but between 2018 and 2019, I'd hit a wall. Real estate has been and always will be my compass, but the noise of the industry was getting to me. I know this because even the small, frivolous lawsuits were starting to annoy me. There was one in Arizona where a guy made his living suing property owners over ADA compliance minutiae. He sued us because our signage wasn't high enough by the new standards. A parking stall was a foot too narrow. We hadn't been neglectful, but the cost of fighting was often higher than settling. That kind of constant nitpicking chips away at one's passion.

At the same time, my kids were fairly young, showing no interest in the business. What was the point of holding onto property for a legacy if they weren't interested in it when I wanted to retire? Real estate cycles are lengthy, because they're tied to broader economic trends—such as interest rates, business cycles, and market demands. All these factors add to the potential for instability. Properties aren't always cash flow positive, and they don't appreciate overnight. They go through phases of growth, stagnation, and sometimes decline, depending on location and timing. Holding onto real estate is a marathon, not a sprint, and it requires patience to realize an investment's full value. The real estate market had been on a bull run since 2010, and I had no desire to wait out the next cycle. If I wasn't prepared to work through the next full cycle, I could be exposed to declining market values and stuck holding the properties, or worse, selling on the decline.

It was time for another turning point in my life: I began selling properties. By sheer luck—or maybe it was timing—I liquidated my holdings before the COVID pandemic gutted retail and other segments of the real estate market. By the time the pandemic hit in March 2020, I only had one retail property left in Billings, Montana. The retail center in Billings was a lesson in leadership. As tenants panicked, I first spoke with my lender and requested a forbearance. Then, I wrote the tenants a letter promising they wouldn't lose their spaces for nonperformance. I wanted the message to be that I had no surprises and was making a recalibration. Yes, I was in business to make money, but I'd rather lose a few months' rent than lose the tenants entirely. These were more than just spaces to rent; these businesses were the foundations upon which many families depended. One tenant left me a voicemail in tears, thanking me for saving her business.

Except for another expansive storage condominium project in Chandler, Arizona, that Shane would manage, I finally sold that last retail property in 2021, during the brief low-interest-rate environment caused by the pandemic, pivoting my career trajectory. Peggy and I turned our full attention once again to managing our portfolio through stock and options trading. It became a family affair—our kids were learning to trade and taking responsibility for their share of what they would inevitably inherit.

Ironically, several years after winding down my real estate career, I noticed something remarkable in Wilson, my youngest. Late one night, we were on the phone discussing a real estate case study he was working on for class at Boston College. I listened as he rattled off comps, analyzed market conditions, and broke down financials with clean understanding. *This kid*, I thought to myself. *He really gets it*.

I don't know if Wilson will follow in my footsteps, but it's comforting to see the spark of understanding in him, the kind that might one day light his path. After all, he comes from a long line of great conversationalists and good listeners.

31

Saint Sophia

Adversity introduces a man to himself.
—Anonymous

Friday Morning, May 3

One of the more uplifting moments of my uneventful, several-day-long ICU stay was meeting Sophia, a nurse who was not only helpful with Peggy but left an indelible mark on me, despite the brevity of our interactions. Sophia was quick to remind me that we had actually met days earlier—back when I was unconscious and unaware of the world around me. I feel like she acted as the true conduit of my before and after moments, from the time I was sedated to my full awakening three days later. During that time, she had interacted extensively with my family—my parents, brothers, kids, and close friends, all of whom were desperate for answers about my precarious condition.

"I met your family—they were so supportive and hopeful," Sophia said with a smile the first time I was cognizant enough to have a conversation with her. Sophia bent the rules for my friends and family, letting more loved ones into my ICU room than was typically allowed. It was surreal to hear her talk about such a personal connection to my family while I had no memory of her at all. However, I quickly realized Sophia had the unique ability to balance the life-and-death stakes of her job with a personal touch that made her patients and their families feel genuinely cared for.

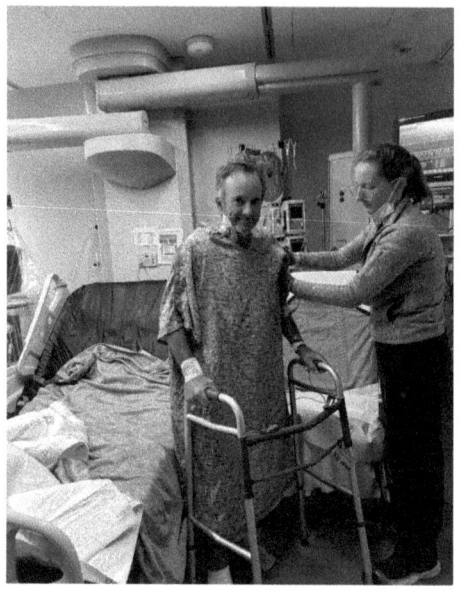

Nurse St. Sophia

Sophia embodied that spirit of total care in any situation by moving with a calm confidence that steadied everyone around her. She had a knack for blending professionalism with genuine warmth, making even the most sterile hospital moments feel a little more human. Whether it was adjusting a monitor or offering Peggy a reassuring smile, I was told Sophia's presence was like a quiet anchor in the storm, reminding us that even in the chaos, care and kindness could still prevail in the face of the unknown.

Sophia helped prepare me for the transition to cardiac recovery—but not without some drama mixed with some humor. That morning, I'd been given a laxative, and my stomach was finally starting to respond. After all, it had been a week since I'd been reminded what "regular" felt like. As Sophia bustled about getting me ready for the move, I asked her to help me to the restroom. Without missing a beat, she suggested a bedpan instead. I hesitated, feeling awkward. We had just met, and this felt like a bridge too far for our fledgling patient-nurse relationship.

"Are you sure?" I asked, eyeing her warily.

"Trust me, John, it's easier this way," she said confidently, her tone leaving little room for debate.

Time was of the essence, so I reluctantly agreed. To ease my embarrassment, I tactfully responded, "Well, you've got a baby at home, so I guess you're used to this sort of thing."

Sophia laughed. "Actually, it's easier with adults. Besides, the sheets are going to the laundry anyway."

That was all the assurance I needed. What followed was, let's say, less than dignified. As the episode unfolded, I found myself apologizing profusely. "This is probably more than you bargained for," I said, mortified.

Sophia waved it off with a smile. "John, this is nothing. I've seen it all." She said I was a success story. Her calm disposition turned what could have been a humiliating moment into one of connection and humanity.

When it was over, I could only muster one last attempt at levity. "If we ever get the boat my wife has promised, you and your husband will be our guests."

Owning a boat was one of the crazy ideas Peggy and I had talked about over the years, but it was even crazier of her to whisper it in my ear during my darkest hour: "If you stay alive, we're going to buy the boat we've always talked about." It was a fantasy that gave us something to look forward to, a reminder that life existed beyond the sterile walls of the hospital. Those imagined moments of freedom felt like an antidote to the machines that hummed around me. It wasn't just about the boat—it was about reclaiming a sense of normalcy, joy, and being untethered from the grips of this medical nightmare.

In speaking with Sophia several months later, she shared some great insights as someone who sees troubling cases day in and day out. She meets a lot of people with broken families or psychosocial issues compounded with health issues. She referenced one of the surgeons, who said, "The body follows the mind." She went on to say: "As soon as John woke up, he had a lot of perspective. He was so lucky and just so grateful to be alive. You can choose to feel this way or choose to be the victim. Maybe that's why he's successful in life—he's that person that looks at the cup as half full."

With my mess cleaned and IVs in tow, Sophia, now crowned Saint Sophia, wheeled me out of the ICU. Compared with the last few days, this was an exciting trek up an elevator and into my new room on the eighth floor. The change was palpable. Gone were the constant hum of monitors and the frenetic energy of the ICU. In its place was a quieter, more subdued, and more isolated environment. I felt a sinking sensation, as if I were leaving behind the safety net of the ICU and entering a new, uncertain chapter. My recovery felt less urgent now but no less daunting.

Friday Afternoon, May 3

Moving from the ICU to a regular cardiac recovery room was a strange kind of letdown; I would have assumed it would feel like a high point, proof that I was finally out of the woods. Don't get me wrong—I was thrilled to leave the intensive care unit. But after fighting for my life, surviving sepsis, cardiac arrest, and multiple surgeries, I was suddenly staring down the long, uncertain road of recovery. The immediate danger had passed, but the path back to anything resembling normalcy had only just begun. For a moment, I truly felt sorry for myself. In some odd way, I missed the constant motion and attention of the ICU, though I only have limited memories—or more like vivid flashes—after the ECMO was removed. I could lose myself and forget about my pain in the constant rush of the ICU.

In the cardiac recovery unit, the focus was understandably on my heart rather than the grotesque damage to my right leg and foot.

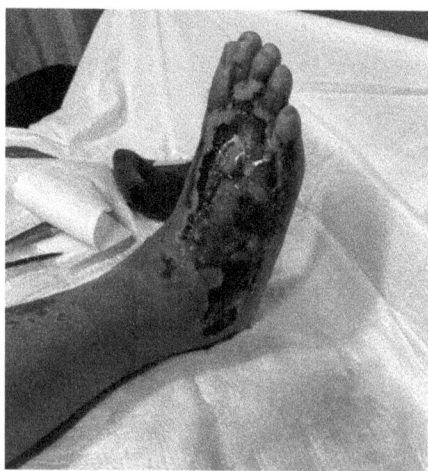

The damage to my right foot from venom and bacteria

If I had been placed on a trauma floor, my limb might have received more attention; instead, I became something of an anomaly to the parade of doctors and nurses who came through to check my cardiac vitals. Each one seemed intrigued by my unique story. "I've reviewed your records," one nurse said. "I've never seen the results of a suspected box jellyfish sting and subsequent sepsis shock before."

Aside from those flurries of activity, the routine in cardiac recovery was monotonous. Unlike the ICU, I didn't have someone helping me get up and move regularly. Most of my interactions revolved around wound care and again pain management—rating it on a scale of 0 to 10 and receiving a corresponding dose of Tylenol, Tramadol, or even Oxycodone. My pain levels hovered between 7 and 8, making even the simplest tasks excruciating. Someone had written on the whiteboard in my room: "Restoring my strength." It was a reminder of my ultimate goal. I don't remember if I'd written it or if a nurse had, but it hung there as a silent motivator. It must have been Blair, because it was also written on the whiteboard that my favorite music was by Taylor Swift. It took me a week or so to notice this factoid right in front of me and must have provided cheap entertainment to the staff as they came and went, not knowing it was something Blair and I shared together.

Physical and occupational therapists visited sporadically, each session feeling like a small mountain to climb. My leg was swollen and looked like a tree trunk, so standing for even a few seconds was unbearable. I relied on a handheld urinal to avoid getting up, only leaving my bed twice a day—once for a more extended trip to use the toilet and once for early morning weigh-in. The daily weight check protocol lasted all of fifteen seconds before I collapsed back onto the bed, seeking relief. I managed a few arm and core exercises with a resistance band, but my motivation was fleeting. In total, I probably worked out just three or four very short times during my stay in cardiac recovery.

Saturday Evening, May 4

For the first time since April 26, I managed to roll onto my left side and lift my swollen right leg onto my left. This night marked a turning point. It was the most comfortable position I'd been in for days. I slept deeply that night, and when I awoke in the early hours the following morning, I had an epiphany. My mind was racing with thoughts of writing not just a health update for friends and family, but something bigger.

By the time my kids arrived for their morning visit, I was bursting to share my idea. Blair had expected me to have the draft of my health update for her to proofread. Instead, I greeted her with a mischievous grin. "Blair, I had an epiphany in the middle of the night."

She rolled her eyes, half-amused, half-concerned. "Oh God, what now?"

"Hear me out," I said, my excitement spilling over. "I think I've decided to write a memoir."

32

Long Road Back

Random question: Why do people say "Be careful" after you trip on the sidewalk?
—Jerry Seinfeld

Tuesday, May 7th

My slow transition from the hospital to a nearby hotel gave us a glimpse of what life might look like outside the hospital. It offered Peggy a chance to resume parts of her daily routine while still caring for me constantly. For me, on the surface, it meant confronting a new set of limitations—learning to walk again, managing wound care, organizing medications, and facing a version of myself I barely recognized. But on a deeper level, seeing the world from that wheelchair altered my perspective in ways I hadn't expected. After years of designing and retrofitting properties to be ADA accessible, I was now the one who needed the ramp, the grab bar, the wider doorway. I've never been more grateful for the presence of a handrail in a public restroom.

Mother's Day was the day I was finally released from CPMC outpatient care. Before flying home, I spent the morning with my mother. Under normal circumstances, we might have gone for a long walk along Crissy Field, maybe stopping at the Warming Hut Park Store for coffee and conversation with the Golden Gate Bridge in view. But this year was different. Instead, we took a slow drive together, checking out familiar corners of the city and noticing what had changed: South Park, the neighborhoods around Dogpatch, places that once held my footprints now seen through a car window.

It was deeply comforting to be with my mother that day. She's always had a quiet way of making things feel okay, even when they're not. But what struck me most, what humbled me, was the role reversal. Instead of me driving my eighty-five-year-old mother, she was the one driving me. That shift said more than either of us could. It was a gentle reminder of how fragile recovery can be, and how even in my weakest moments, I was still being cared for with love that spanned a lifetime.

Returning home to Sun Valley turned out to be a brief and difficult visit. That first attempt at reintegration was far from the hopeful homecoming I had imagined. I wasn't ready to see friends or make conversation. I wasn't physically strong enough for full rehab or emotionally prepared for normal life. It was mostly quiet hours resting, adjusting, and trying to understand what healing at home would require.

The wound care team at St. Luke's in Hailey was prepared to receive me, but after just five days, they became alarmed by the worsening condition of my foot. The threat of infection loomed too large. On May 17, wound care specialist Dr. Barns and the nurse practitioner Mandy gently told us our options: seek more specialized care in Boise or return to CPMC in San Francisco. We chose the latter, finding a strange sense of comfort in going back to the place that had already seen us through the worst. It wasn't what we had hoped for, but it felt familiar, and that counted for something.

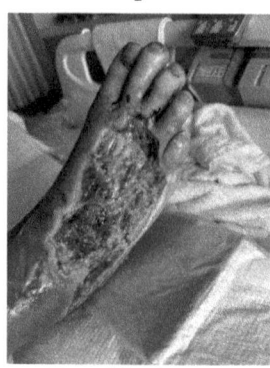

Post debridement of my right foot

Back at CPMC, a plastic surgeon named Dr. Parrett had taken my case from Dr. Kind and was monitoring my condition remotely. Through daily images, he had already concluded that the next step would be a full debridement of the top section of my foot. To my surprise, he didn't wait; he booked the first available operating room: 7:00 a.m. on Sunday morning, May 19. Just like that, surgery number four was underway.

Heart of the Journey

This time, it came with something new: a wound vacuum. It was not exactly a medical device I ever imagined becoming familiar with, but it quickly became central to my recovery. The wound vacuum works by removing fluids and infection from the affected area, helping stimulate new tissue growth and speed healing. In my case, it would eventually connect to multiple sites on my right leg.

Picture an octopus clinging to my leg, its tentacles transformed into tubes, pulling blood and fluid from each wound into a small, humming machine I carried with me. It stayed with me during five more days of recovery in the hospital, and then, like so much of this unexpected journey, it came with me—first to San Diego and then home to Sun Valley.

A major goal that kept me going was attending Hayden's graduation from the University of San Diego on May 26. We arranged for special seating to accommodate my mobility issues. I was determined to be there, to see him walk across that stage. Blair remembered watching me inch downstairs with my little knee scooter, slow and awkward but unstoppable. Maneuvering wasn't easy, but there was no chance I was going to miss celebrating that weekend with my family.

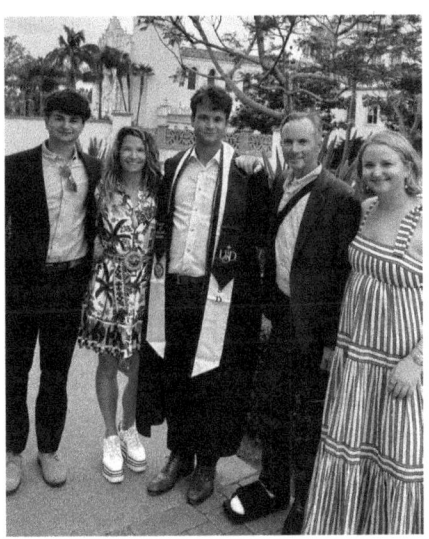

**Hayden's graduation from
University of San Diego, May 2024**

The surgery ushered in a parade of unfamiliar routines, devices, and discomforts—most notably the wound vacuum system, which became a constant presence in our lives. It required daily attention and frequent adjustments, especially at night, when the tubing would twist around me, disrupting my sleep and adding fatigue to my frustration. Still, it was essential, helping to regenerate tissue and heal the raw surface left behind by the debridement.

Social outings—as much as I craved them—required careful planning. When I ventured into town with friends, I found discreet ways to manage my wound vac. Instead of just slinging it over my shoulder and letting the world stare, I got a little crafty: I ran the medical cords down my pant leg and carried the device like a purse. Oddly enough, the machine seemed to have a sense of humor—or maybe we just needed one. It would occasionally let out an embarrassing "farting" noise, adding a touch of unintentional comedy to otherwise heavy moments. It gave us something to laugh about when we needed it most.

Our bedroom slowly transformed into something closer to an infirmary. I slept on a separate mattress on the floor, leg elevated, machine and pills at my side. Peggy, a light and sensitive sleeper, had to adjust to the persistent hum and unpredictable sounds, while still tending to my every need. Even something as simple as using the bathroom became a careful production. I relied on a portable urinal at night to avoid the risk of tripping while dragging the wound vacuum behind me.

Amid the disruption, I found pockets of rest thanks to gabapentin, which helped dull the pain and quiet the nerve spasms that would occasionally flash like lightning through my foot. Those sensations were sharp, sudden, and terrifying, physical echoes of just how far my body had fallen and how far I still had to go.

It was deeply frustrating to be so dependent on Peggy for nearly everything—wound care, driving, ordering supplies, meals—while she was trying to reclaim even fragments of her own life. I could sense her weariness, especially when I didn't follow every instruction to the letter, or when I was hesitant to embrace every alternative therapy presented to us: hyperbaric chambers, acupuncture, massage, and even a device called a BEMER machine, which was supposed to stimulate vascular circulation. I often felt like I was being bombarded with suggestions, pulled in every direction by competing ideas about how to heal faster.

But I knew my own body, and I trusted it. Time, not magic, was what I needed. I wasn't chasing a shortcut. And, truthfully, I've never liked taking pills, herbal or pharmaceutical, and there were too many of both. Add to that the tangle of tubes from the wound vacuum machine, tethered to me day and night, and it was all more than just physically exhausting. Showers were out of the question. Every task became an ordeal. I did my best to go with the flow, but there were moments I wanted to scream, "Enough!"

Somewhere during this stretch, it hit me: Between wound care appointments, we were essentially "cowboying" this whole thing on our own. We had expert doctors in their respective fields, but no one overseeing the whole picture, no single advocate for my recovery. Peggy, with unrelenting dedication, was trying to perform sterile bandage changes on our family room couch. We were sending off photos to my plastic surgeon, Dr. Parrett in San Francisco, and the wound care team in Hailey, then waiting for texts or emails with instructions. It felt like we were improvising every single day.

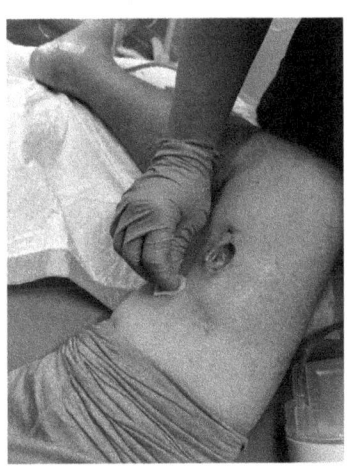

More mysterious toxins releasing from my right leg during recovery

Each wound had its own shifting protocol. The two on my right leg—open, raw holes—seemed to be releasing whatever venom or bacteria remained in my system. We had to stuff them daily with a shoelace-like material soaked in antiseptic, pushing it in as deep as possible to avoid infection before carefully covering them. My foot required the more technical wound vacuum, which came with its own set of challenges and complications.

And yet, somehow, progress came— slow, hard-fought, but real. Each stage of recovery was a small triumph. Transitioning from wheelchair to walker was an emotional milestone. I remember the pride of navigating our house with the walker, step by shaky step. Soon, I could walk part of the driveway and back—then, after a few days, down the driveway, around the street, and back up again. It felt huge.

Of course, the road wasn't smooth. My right foot required yet another procedure, surgery number five, scheduled for June 10 in San Francisco. This time it was a skin graft, taken from my right thigh, to cover the debrided area that was ready for new skin. It was an unsettling process. The graft introduced new complications: persistent swelling, inflammation, and a renewed need for elevation and compression. It was disheartening. After all my close calls—sepsis, cardiac arrest, and multiple surgeries—I had somehow emerged without lasting damage to my heart or organs. And yet, it was my foot and skin graft that were holding me hostage, the same foot that had been sliced open in the ICU as an emergency measure to relieve the swelling and pressure at the very start of this ordeal.

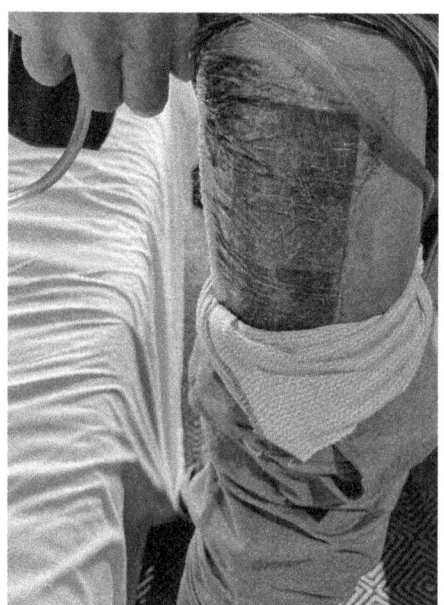

The fifth and final surgery, taking skin from my thigh and grafting onto my foot

Heart of the Journey

Humor, once again, proved to be the antidote that carried us through. On June 15, almost eight weeks after this ordeal began, Peggy and I left Dr. Parrett's office on Webster Street in San Francisco after being cleared yet again, this time carrying the wound vacuum neatly packed in a box, ready to return to the company that had rented it to us. As fate would have it, an iconic brown UPS truck turned the corner just as we stepped outside. We looked at each other and instantly had the same thought: Let's flag him down and finally get this machine out of our lives. Once the box was gone, without a word, we kissed each other, a spontaneous moment of joy, relief, and quiet triumph. It wasn't just a return; it was a milestone. A small but mighty victory.

***

The day I was cleared to drive, June 20, 2024, represented another pivotal milestone. It signaled a reclaiming of independence that had been stripped away by my condition. No longer reliant on others for transportation, I could begin reestablishing some semblance of my former routines.

While the months of recovery are a necessary part of my personal story, I acknowledge that they placed an inevitable strain on family relationships, particularly between Peggy and me. As Blair once observed, "Both my parents are very independent. Now, Mom suddenly has to stay home to take care of Dad. He can't do anything. He can't go anywhere, and he has all these wound care and physical therapy appointments."

There was a quiet tug-of-war unfolding between my instinct to fight for independence and my growing need to surrender to help. I wrestled with frustration at my own limitations, even as I tried to make peace with them. Peggy, meanwhile, bore the weight of the household and my care. At the same time, I knew the role of full-time caregiver wasn't one she had signed up for. I recognized this tension and tried to make conscious efforts to minimize the burden on her, though at times it felt like an emotional balancing act neither of us had trained for.

There was another quiet surrender at play, one that didn't involve words, just the slow unraveling of what I thought the next few months would be.

Swimming was uncertain, the Scotland golf trip was off the table, and a fall hiking trek through the Alps was postponed at my doctors' strong advice. I was not one to resign myself, but the challenge was clearly too large to overcome. Sitting there, I realized I'd need to come up with a different kind of pursuit, one that matched my new limitations but still gave me purpose.

***

While it would have been easy and understandable to isolate myself during recovery, I found ways to maintain social connections on my own terms. I needed my community of friends and some sense of normalcy. So, I established a daily routine of hosting friends for lunch on my favorite part of our patio at home. It overlooks our flower garden with a fantastic view of Bald Mountain.

Soon, I had this great thing going, due to the many caring friendships in the valley. I'd say, "Thank you so much for reaching out. I'd love to see you. How about tomorrow at noon?"

They'd often ask, "Can I bring lunch?" The answer was always yes.

During these gatherings, I channeled my grandmother Terry's wisdom and made a conscious effort to focus on my friends' lives rather than my medical situation. If they didn't know about the accident, I would give them the nitty-gritty overview, but otherwise, I just tried to get back to relationships, friendships, and doing things that made me happy.

In our tight-knit community, news of my medical crisis had spread widely. On July 27, I took my first trail walk on Proctor Mountain behind our home. I placed a bandage over my open wound to provide a cushion from chafing and prevent further injury. On the trail, I was stopped six times by concerned acquaintances who had heard about my incident—a true testament to the community of friends we've been fortunate to be part of in Sun Valley for the past several decades. The only significant sporting activity I reclaimed early in August was a round of golf, although in a modified form. Using a cart instead of walking the course, I found I could still swing well, despite my foot limitations.

***

Heart of the Journey

Golf has always held a special place in my heart—a passion my father and I have shared for as long as I can remember. We've played memorable rounds together, from the World Father–Son Golf Tournament in Waterville, Ireland, to the rugged beauty of Bandon Dunes, Oregon, to leisurely walks down the fairways of the San Francisco Golf Club.

For my father, giving back to the sport all began in 1993, when a friend encouraged him to attend a rules school. He took to it quickly, developing such a deep knowledge of the game that he began officiating Northern California Golf Association (NCGA) tournaments. During his time as president of the NCGA Foundation, he grew concerned about the financial barriers preventing many kids from accessing the game. Looking for a meaningful way to give back, he and a group of like-minded cofounders devised a plan: offer youth ages six to eighteen the opportunity to play golf for just five dollars a round. They called the initiative Youth on Course.

Since then, the organization has subsidized millions of golf rounds for young players across the United States and Canada. My father's lifelong dedication to the game and its community has left a powerful mark on junior golf, a legacy that continues to grow. It's an achievement admired by all who know him, and one that fills our family with deep pride.

For me, golf has always been more than competition or scorecards. It's been a steady thread woven through my life, deepening friendships and connecting me to something larger than myself. The relationships I've built on the course—many lasting decades—are among the most meaningful I've known. There's something about the shared challenges, quiet competition, and banter that forges lasting bonds and a wealth of unforgettable memories.

***

2008 was the year I first came across a guy named Rob McGowan. He moved over from Los Angeles to Sun Valley with the same lifestyle dreams we all had at the time. He was part of a ragtag group of golfers with whom we both connected. He stood out to me because he was using a 4-iron on the tee box instead of a driver. He clearly stated, "I'm struggling with this driver." This was endearing, as it's still the case today, more than fifteen years later. What began as a few casual rounds of golf while watching the markets drop in 2008 evolved into hours of uninterrupted time and travel together—time where we could talk about everything from business, to parenting, to our deepest personal struggles. There's not a topic that's off-limits between us.

Rob is often the voice of reason—not just for me, but for those with whom he chooses to surround himself. He's the type of friend who will speak up on touchy topics of loyalty, judgment, and morality because he cares enough to be honest, not because he wants to critique. He is known in his circles to have impeccable taste. We have a running joke about there being two ways to do things: "Rob's way and the wrong way." The truth is, I've come to trust his judgment deeply over the years—and most importantly, we've always had each other's backs as loyal wingmen. Rob and I have famously traveled together to many remarkable golf destinations around the U.S., Ireland, Scotland, and Italy. We like to think of ourselves as the modern-day Lewis and Clark—explorers of life's great unknowns, carefully documenting exotic flora, elusive fauna, and any decent coffee shops along our way.

Rob introduced me some time ago to a man named Steve Miner, who happened to be a movie director from Los Angeles. He and I played golf on occasion. As we stood on the first tee at Los Angeles Country Club South, I politely asked what the wager for the round would be. To my surprise, he said he wasn't interested in playing for money. I pressed a little, offering this: "How about if I lose, I'll pay you twenty dollars—but if I win, Blair gets a walk-on role in your latest TV series, *Switched at Birth*?" We'd been watching it as a family and knew he was directing the popular ABC Family series. To my amazement, he agreed. "That works for me," he said.

There are certain moments in golf you just don't forget. It was a close and spirited match from the start. We traded the lead throughout the round, still tied through the 16th hole. We both bogeyed the 17th hole, keeping it even heading into the 18th—a 428-yard par four. We each found the fairway with solid drives. My second shot landed about twenty feet from the pin. Steve needed two more to reach the green, meaning he'd have to sink a long putt to match my two-putt par. He struck his putt with confidence—it tracked well but caught the edge and lipped out. A tap-in bogey wasn't enough. I had won the match. He took the loss like a gentleman, and soon after, plans were made to get Blair to L.A.

Several months later, at Steve's invitation, we drove to a nondescript warehouse in Santa Clarita, California. It was beyond exciting to watch Blair beam with confidence—Steve even had a dressing trailer with her name on the door. Being on set was fascinating and gave me a deep appreciation for everything that goes into filming. I stood behind the director, watching my young daughter on camera, mingling with seasoned adult actors. Even though it was just a brief cameo, the experience was worth far more than the twenty-dollar wager. It was priceless.

***

Thankfully, my physical limitations at the time didn't restrict my golf in any meaningful way. It provided not just limited exercise but also necessary social reconnection. Swimming, however, required some creative adaptations. With an open wound that couldn't get wet, I placed a vacuum bag over my foot when entering pools. I could use my arms and swim aggressively, but not my legs. Still, the modifications allowed me to regain another of my favorite activities.

Each small step forward helped me feel like normalcy was just around the corner. And each activity required careful risk assessment and medical clearance. Some doctors advised extreme caution; one vascular surgeon recommended canceling the upcoming European trip entirely, fearing I'd be too active and cause a setback in healing. But I found ways to balance cautious activities with living the life I wanted. As I prepared for hiking in the Alps in early September, my approach was simple: do everything, but do it lightly—light hiking, light swimming, light walking, and light eating, too.

Four months into recovery, I acknowledged that true normal still remained elusive. My foot still functioned at maybe 80 percent of its capacity, and I continued to experience limitations. Instead of being frustrated that I wasn't back to 100 percent, I accepted where I was. The concept of a "new normal" gradually replaced my expectations of returning to my pre-illness state. The persistent post-trauma edema in my leg, commonly known as swelling, would unfortunately continue well past a year from the incident. I determined I would be thankful for each day, and gracious with myself as I continued on the long road back.

33

Life Saga

*Life is not measured by the number of breaths we take,
but by the moments that take our breath away.*
—Maya Angelou

Throughout recovery, I maintained an upbeat attitude that surprised those around me. Sure, there had been little annoyances here and there, but I was always quick to remember how close I'd come to a fate far worse than an injured foot. That gave me the patience to slow down, take a deep breath, and be grateful for what I could do. This wasn't mere positivity but a deliberate philosophical stance. I like to believe that I'm a lucky person to get through all this and that I have a great supportive family and friend group.

This experience also fundamentally shifted my perspective on risk. As an adventurous spirit who formerly embraced physical challenges and tackled my fears head-on, I found myself more cautious post-recovery not necessarily out of fear but wisdom. I'm noticing I'm grabbing onto more handrails as I walk downstairs—some of it is the caution of age, and some of it is the reality that I don't want to slip.

This new risk assessment has extended beyond physical activities to everyday decisions. When I cross the street now, I look twice. I used to drift through stop signs if there were no other people around. Now, I stop like I should; I think they call people like me law-abiding citizens. The extra five seconds I would have gained by rolling through instead of fully stopping aren't going to make a difference in my day.

This experience also deepened my emotional connections. I find myself more openly expressing appreciation for relationships, especially with Peggy and my children. I say "I love you" more, both to family and friends, which is different from how I was raised. I give more hugs. I'm more present in conversations, and I've become a better listener and a more patient friend, husband, and father.

It's interesting that when it comes to parenting, most people model how they were raised and feel that's how the next generation should do things. As a parent, I once believed this to be true as well. It's taken until recently for me to be accepting of the way my kids (and the next generation as a whole) decide to lead their lives.

My relationship with Peggy has been strengthened in unexpected ways. She has even gone so far as to say that writing this book has made up for sixty years of therapy I never had. As retired empty nesters, I look forward to more traveling with her and sharing new experiences.

With our independent adult children and my urgent medical needs in the past, we can focus more on just the two of us, reconnecting and strengthening our love and friendship. To be able to share your life with somebody through the adventures—and this certainly was an adventure—is a gift.

With this second chance at life, I've come to understand more deeply the ripple effects our choices and conversations have on those we love. I'm able to savor the time with others, whereas before, there were times I took my close relationships for granted. I now carry a greater sense of accountability, both to myself and to those around me.

My relationship with time has shifted, too. Before, I measured success in sub-80 golf scores, business deals, and marathon finish times. Now, I think more about what I call QTR—Quality Time Remaining. It's not about counting down days but making each one matter, though that doesn't mean every moment needs to be extraordinary. Sometimes, the most meaningful days are spent reading on the couch or tending to my bees. The satisfaction comes not from what I'm doing but from being present enough to fully experience it alone or with people I love.

That truth hit home like never before a few months into my recovery, when Peggy's first cousin, Joel Barnett, suddenly grabbed me by the collar and, with emotion in his voice, demanded, "Don't you ever do that to us again!"

***

People often ask if I'm angry about what happened or if I feel like a victim. The truth is, I don't. This experience wasn't something that happened *to* me—it was something that happened *for* me. That might sound like motivational poster wisdom, but there's profound truth in it. The ocean has always been both my fear and my challenge. That Tuesday morning swim was a choice I made, knowing the risks but believing in the rewards. I wouldn't change that decision, even knowing the outcome. If anything, this event has given me the opportunity to meet some incredible doctors and nurses who truly exemplify the mission of saving lives while continuing to engage in groundbreaking research.

Questions still lingered for me as to the underlying cause of how I contracted sepsis. I was able to coordinate a meeting in the Hawaiian Islands on August 5, with a renowned expert on infectious disease and marine envenomation, Dr. Jonathan Dworkin. Peggy and I already had plans to return to the islands, so this in-person meeting was a timely and fortunate opportunity to speak directly with someone whose insights could bring both clarity and peace of mind after months of uncertainty.

After discussing my case and looking over the records, he believed the only reasonable conclusion for what happened to me was that I had group A streptococcus (strep A) and a delayed release of toxins from the jellyfish sting that resulted in the sepsis. Bacteria and toxins had colonized my inflamed skin and crawled into my body from the sting, a small cut, or both, which had led to my streptococcal toxic shock syndrome (STSS) and subsequent organ failures. Hearing Dr. Dworkin's assessment was a strange mix of both relief and reckoning—relief at finally having a plausible, science-backed explanation added to other speculations, but also a sobering sense of awe at how close I had come to the edge from something so deceptively simple.

I also kept in touch with my cardiologist, Dr. Daniels, who remains outspoken in his diagnosis of an envenomation event from a box jellyfish, specifically Irukandji syndrome. He was so convinced that he wrote about my case in a cardiac medical journal. Dr. Daniels thinks the delayed reaction of the venom—and the fact that I didn't die—can be attributed to my overall good physical health and conditioning. I will always be in debt to him and his sharp ability to assess and act on my condition so quickly. His passion for cardiology and saving lives runs deep. He cares not only for the cardiac patient but for improving the medical system as a whole. He dedicates whatever spare time he has to advanced devices that improve patients' lives during and after surgery.

The renowned biochemist and physiologist Dr. Angel Yanagihara, whose groundbreaking research focuses on jellyfish venom and its effects on the human body, has found that there are approximately 4,000 species of jellyfish floating around the world's oceans. Most of those are relatively harmless, and their stings are no worse than wasp or bee stings, like the ones I'd previously encountered before the Hawaii incident.

However, the fifty-ish species of box jellyfish are a different story. Box jellyfish tentacles have hundreds of thousands of specialized cells that shoot microscopic, venom-filled harpoons into their victims. The absorption rate of the venom, as well as the characteristics of the venom itself, varies wildly from species to species, as well as how the victim might react.

I have continued to be in awe of these doctors, who were still invested in my case and healing journey. I can only hope that if they ever encounter another victim of a box jellyfish sting, my case will have given them additional knowledge and a more streamlined guide on how to treat their patients for the best chance of success.

***

One of the beautiful opportunities to result from my accident has been reconnecting with friends. It had been several decades since we'd been in touch, but Greg Applegarth, the childhood friend I'd known since Stuart Hall Grammar School and previously worked with at the Pi Phi sorority house at Berkeley, reappeared in my life completely out of the blue in the form of a handwritten letter I received once I was back home and healing. Greg was the only distant person in my life to reach out in such a personal way. He expressed concern, offered support, and wished me well. It was a gesture that touched me deeply. I hadn't spoken to Greg in years, but there he was. He had taken the time to write.

After reading Greg's note, I took a moment to reflect on the significance of connection and prioritizing purpose over pleasure. His example of thoughtful friendship was a reminder to be present for the people who matter, even when life becomes overwhelming.

Then there is another friend and cherished confidant, Andy Mack, whom I met in Hawaii years earlier. Andy checked in on me several times during my recovery and once said, "Life moves quickly when you hit your fifties and sixties. You start counting sunsets and treasuring moments differently." I'm grateful that my brush with mortality has only reinforced these words and the importance of connections with people like Andy, who remind you what friendship truly means. From the day we met, he has been one of my most consistently thoughtful friends in the truest sense of the word—exemplified by his generously helping Johnny Bees Honey get started with beekeeper supplies.

I recall the first moment Andy and I met after passing each other on the pool deck. What started as a polite gesture of hello turned into a fifteen-minute exchange. Since then, we have shared dolphin and whale encounters, a surprise COVID visit in Florida, and, most importantly, endless conversations over our regularly scheduled calls, as he has since relocated to Florida. His wife, Nancy, would often remind us to "stay out of the weeds," which was a soft reminder to not be too critical of certain matters; we truly believe that between the two of us, we have it all figured out.

Our friendship continues to deepen as we discuss everything from politics to current events, toys, and travel. It's one of those rare connections where time and distance don't seem to matter as we solve the world's problems. I would be remiss not to mention that he has the ability to remember things I didn't even know I'd forgotten.

***

The recovery process, while frustrating at times, has offered unexpected gifts: deeper relationships, a newfound appreciation for life's fragility, and a chance to reflect on a life well-lived. I have remained determined not to let my recovery be all-consuming, taking wisdom from my grandmother Terry, who had disdain for elderly friends who only discussed their ailments.

I don't want to be known as the guy defined by his medical events. I don't want them to be the reason my swimming kick isn't what it used to be—or the excuse for skipping the next great hike. Instead, I've chosen to frame the experience in a different light: *Look at all the good that's come from it.*

Certainly, writing this memoir is at the top of that list. My long recovery gave me the time and focus to bring this book to life, something I had only dreamed of achieving. Along the way, it has helped me make sense of life, gain perspective, and, in the process, create a compelling story for others to enjoy—one that I hope offers insight into life, love, luck, risk, and chance.

As I think about my future travel adventures, my foot is still healing but my spirit remains bright. I continue to embody resilience in its truest form. The scars, both physical and emotional, will always remain, but they have become part of a larger story of growth, gratitude, and an evolving understanding of what truly matters.

When I woke up in that hospital bed, tethered to machines and unable to speak, I couldn't have known how profoundly those three lost days would reshape my perspective. The immediate aftermath was focused on survival and recovery—learning to walk again, managing pain, and rebuilding strength. But the deeper changes, the ones that truly matter, emerged gradually in the months that followed.

The *real* transformation hasn't been physical, though my right foot still bears the scars of that encounter. Instead, it's been in how I approach each day. The long road back to full healing still continues, but the journey itself holds unexpected value. In the end, I believe this detour ultimately led to a deeper appreciation of the path.

***

Heart of the Journey

As the morning sun peeks over the Hawaiian mountains, I slip into my white beekeeping suit. My children's words from two years ago still echo in my mind: *Okay, Dad. You said in your retirement this would be one of your hobbies. Let's see it.* They had presented me with a book and a Johnny Bees logo for the honey jars, challenging me to turn my longtime fascination with bees into a reality.

Now, as I approach my stack of hive boxes nestled among the tropical flowering trees and coconut palms, a sense of peace washes over me. The gentle humming of about 65,000 bees going about their daily work fills the air. These aren't just any bees; they're my partners in creating something special, gathering nectar from the diverse Hawaiian flora to produce Johnny Bees Honey, my delicious new hobby.

I've always been drawn to adventure, from rock climbing to ocean swimming, but this is a different kind of adventure—one where the risk comes not from heights or waves, but from thousands of tiny insects that many people instinctively fear. I smile, thinking how I've gone from being a kid who would swat at bees to becoming their devoted keeper.

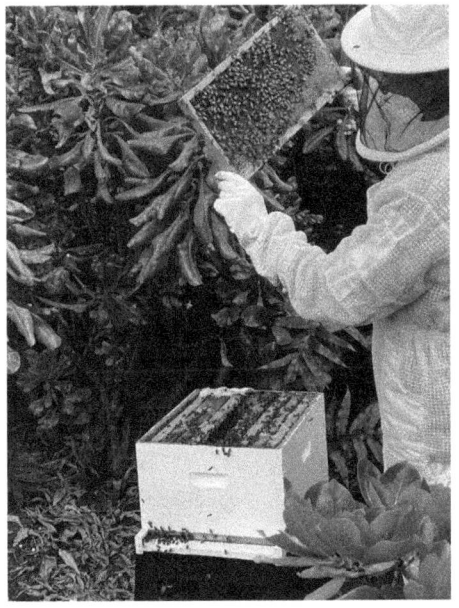

Hawaiian hive inspection

After smoking the hive, I can carefully remove some of the frames. I watch as the bees continue their work, completely unbothered by my presence. The morning light catches the amber honey stored in perfect hexagonal cells. This isn't just about producing honey; it's about finding joy in offering nature's bounty to others. I get to share the bees' honey with so many friends and family—liquid gold harvested gently from the hive and captured in glass jars labelled Johnny Bees.

After checking the frames and ensuring the queen is healthy, I close up the hive. In less than two years, I've joined what the local beekeepers call the "hundred-pound club," producing over a hundred pounds—about twelve gallons—of honey in the last year and half. Each harvest is a testament to the incredible work of my bees in Hawaii's year-round foraging environment. But the true measure of success isn't in the pounds of honey harvested. It's in the satisfaction of nurturing these remarkable insects and giving their gifts to our community.

As I head from the yard back to the house, I reflect on how different this is from my previous career in commercial real estate investment. There's no ROI spreadsheet for the joy of beekeeping, no profit margin to calculate. Sometimes, the sweetest returns in life can't be measured in dollars and cents. In real estate retirement, I've discovered that my most meaningful days are no longer about closing big deals or managing properties but about the simple things in life like tending to my bees.

Taking off my beekeeping suit, I smile. My kids were right to challenge me. What started as a retirement hobby has become something far more significant—a sweet reminder that life's greatest adventures sometimes come in unexpected packages, even in the form of 65,000 tiny, buzzing friends.

Just before I walk into the house, I see the neighborhood cat lounging in a shady part of the garden. To this day, I'm not sure if she belongs to someone or lucked into living her feral life here. When the cat lets us know it's time to feed her, Peggy obliges. It's clear she prefers Peggy over me, which is fine. I've never been much of a cat person, though I have to admit, this cat is growing on me.

The cat's favorite place is a historic outrigger canoe that is prominently displayed in the yard. I feel the canoe has a spiritual connection to the Tahitian culture that found its way by sea to Hawaii. The romantic in me thinks the cat can somehow feel that connection, and that's why she spends so much time there. More than likely, the canoe is just a good vantage point and provides shade and comfort. Most days, that's all you really need.

The wonderful thing about Hawaii is that every day feels like the day before—a perfect tropical day. You wake up and throw on a pair of shorts, a T-shirt, and flip-flops to go about your business. The temperature is mild, and the culture in our community is generally casual. Rarely is there a need to dress up. We are part of a community that has a strong sense of aloha, with a commitment to respect and preserve the local culture and natural environment.

We don't use cars to get around the property. Instead, we rely on electric golf carts, all uniquely named. One of ours is called Mauna Ohana, Hawaiian words that mean "Our Mountain Family." I can say without a doubt that this community has become family to us as well. These relationships run deep.

Family has always been central to my life, but now, I see those connections with new clarity. Watching Blair intuitively complete my written thoughts in the hospital, feeling Hayden's quiet strength as he sat beside me, or witnessing Wilson's unwavering optimism with his message of "You got this, Dad"—these moments revealed dimensions of my children I might have missed in my previous rush through life. And there's Peggy, whose resilience and adaptation to my temporary silence in those early days reminded me why we've weathered every storm together.

Friends tell me I've become more sentimental. They're right. I'm quicker to express appreciation and more intentional about nurturing relationships that matter. Not in grand gestures, but in small acknowledgments of the people who make life rich.

Perhaps the most unexpected change has been in how I view success. Golf, once an obsession, has become an amenity—a way to connect rather than compete. The same goes for my approach to business. I still love the challenge, but I no longer need to prove anything.

This experience isn't a crutch or an excuse. It's simply part of my story. When people hear what happened, they often expect me to have had some profound spiritual awakening or to have completely reinvented myself. The reality is both simpler and more complex. I'm still me, just with a deeper appreciation for life's nuances and a clearer sense of what truly matters.

Looking ahead, I'm not focused on completing a bucket list or racing against time. Instead, I'm building what I hope will be a lasting legacy through the relationships I nurture and the stories I share. Writing this memoir hasn't just been about documenting three lost days. It allowed me to understand how those days changed everything that came after. Those missing days reframed how I see the world, my family, and myself. Most importantly, they taught me that while we can't control what happens to us, *we can control what we do with what happens to us.*

As I write these words, we're planning our next travel adventure—a different kind of journey from our earlier escapades but no less meaningful. Life has a way of presenting new chapters, just when we think we know the whole story. While my brush with mortality hasn't made me fear death, it has taught me to embrace life more fully. Not just the grand moments, but the quiet ones, too. The sweet buzz of bees in my apiary, the laughter around our dinner table, the familiar comfort of Peggy's presence—these are the treasures I might have overlooked before.

Someone recently asked me if I believe in fate, pointing out that a boat we're considering buying is named *Life Saga*. I had to smile at the coincidence. Whether by design or chance, that name captures what I've come to understand: Our lives are made up of ongoing stories, always unfolding. The real adventure isn't in the dramatic plot twists—it's in how we choose to write the next chapter.

So here I am, continuing my saga with a deeper appreciation for every page. I'm not just surviving—I'm thriving, growing, and remaining open to whatever lessons life has yet to teach.

Those three lost days didn't end my story. They gave it new meaning.

And for that, I am profoundly grateful.

The End

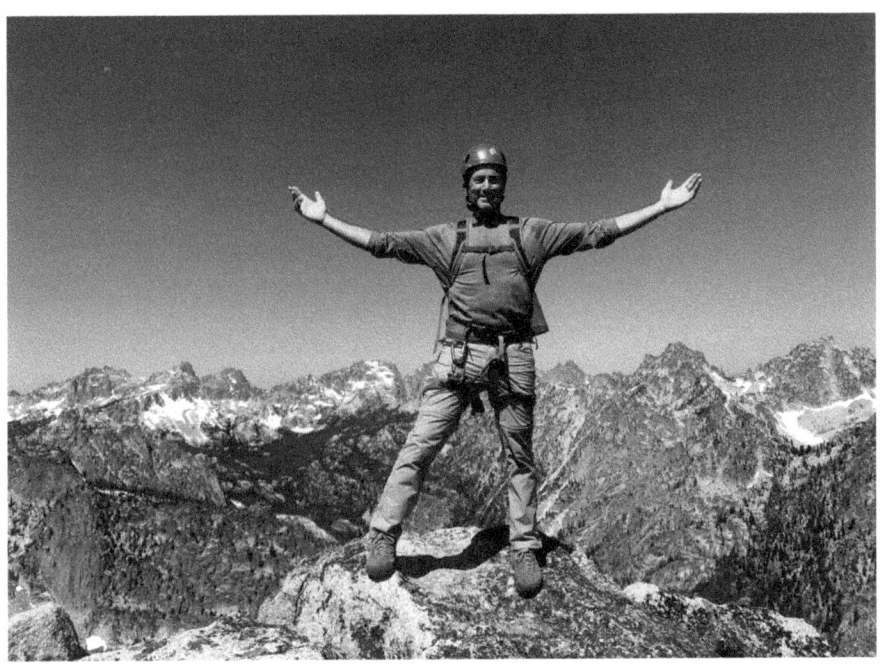
Top of the world

Acknowledgments

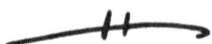

I'm certain that without the love and support of my three children, I might not be here today. Each of them, in their own unique way, inspired this memoir and gave me the courage to tell my story.

Blair offered unwavering encouragement and ultimately became the heartbeat of this book.

Hayden's adventurous spirit opened my eyes to new, less-traveled roads—writing this memoir being one of them.

Wilson has been a motivating soul, often sounding like a wiser, better version of myself, pushing me to keep going.

Peggy—my partner in every way—whose sharp memory and devotion to accuracy kept this project honest and on track. She remains my pillar of strength and the steady light through all of life's chapters.

My parents, Bruce and Barbara, and my brothers, Wayne and Chris, along with Aunt Joan and Stan Green—thank you for your unwavering love and care.

Deidre Grubb, who dropped everything to be there as a true sister to Peggy.

The friends who took the time to visit—Beau Giannini, Bronwyn, Brunner, Renee Goddard, Pat Devlin and Scott Lucas—your presence brought comfort.

I'm deeply grateful to Alice Sullivan for breathing new life into this memoir. Her thoughtful engagement and intuitive understanding helped me discover the voice from within.

Thanks to Michael McConnell, Drew Smith, and Emily Sharp for their editorial expertise, which shaped and refined these pages with care and clarity.

Frank Ewert from Work with Words with his keen eye was able to provide professional editorial guidance. He identified necessary thematic thoughts and, in turn, created a broader reader appeal.

To Dr. Jim Savage for being on-call when it was needed most.

To CPMC and the outstanding medical team: Dr. David Daniels, Dr. Gabriel Kind, Dr. Brian Parrett, Michael Abel, Dr. Shamiq Zackria, Dr. Guy Lubliner, Dr. Adam Simons, Dr. Phillip Kennedy, Dr. Ray Ranjan—and, of course, Sophia Reed, RN.

To Dr. Peter Callander, whose insight, dedication, and friendship I continue to value.

To Dr. Tom Archie, for his foresight and care as my direct primary care provider in the Wood River Valley.

And to the St. Luke's Hailey wound care team: Dr. Randy Barnes, MD, Mandy Allaire, NP, Meghan, and Alison.

About the Authors

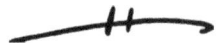

John Baker is an entrepreneur, lifelong adventurer, and father of three whose life has been shaped by both bold pursuits and quiet revelations. From biking across New Zealand in the 1980s to surviving a life-altering medical crisis, his journey has been anything but ordinary. He brings a sharp eye for detail and a deep appreciation for life's subtleties to his writing. A fifth-generation San Franciscan, John met his beloved wife there before the two made their home together in Sun Valley, Idaho, in 1997.

The idea for this memoir came to him in the stillness of night, just after his release from the ICU. "Blair, I had an epiphany last night," he told his daughter with a mischievous grin.

She rolled her eyes. "Oh God. What now?"

His reply: "I think I've decided to write a memoir." That spark became the first step toward this deeply personal reflection on resilience, gratitude, and the surprising ways in which our greatest trials illuminate what matters most.

Blair Baker is a lifelong book lover who's always working toward her nearly impossible yearly reading goal. Blair currently lives in New York City but is known to pop up on her parents' globe-trotting adventures whenever there's a good reason (or a nice hotel). She is grateful for the opportunity to write the foreword for this book, but more than anything, she is grateful that her dad is here today to share his story with you.

Alice Sullivan is a #1 bestselling *Wall Street Journal* ghostwriter, *New York Times* bestselling editor (11 times over), collaborator, and speaker. An avid storyteller, she has written 65 books and edited over 1,300 titles since 2001. She specializes in memoir because she loves stories of triumph, determination, and personal reflection.